HELP YOURSELF

—————— TO ——————

BETTER HEALTH

WHILE TAKING LONG TERM MEDICATION

DOUGLAS HICKS

ISBN: 979-8-89031-655-4 (sc)
ISBN: 979-8-89031-656-1 (hc)
ISBN: 979-8-89031-657-8 (e)

Because of the dynamic nature of the Internet, any web addresses or links contained in this book may have changed since publication and may no longer be valid. The views expressed in this work are solely those of the author and do not necessarily reflect the views of the publisher, and the publisher hereby disclaims any responsibility for them.

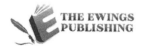

THE EWINGS PUBLISHING

One Galleria Blvd., Suite 1900, Metairie, LA 70001
(504) 702-6708

CONTENTS

AUTHOR'S DISCLOSURE AND NOTICE TO THE READER

The experiences and findings expressed in this book are my own. They are the result of my own real life events. No university or other third party has trained me in any of the subjects herein. Where relevant, I have referred to the supporting work and products of others whose work, findings, and products have, and continue to, benefit my health and vitality. Each of us is unique, and you may find that your response to the recommendations may vary from my own. I'm a Mr Average sharing my findings and story with the aim of helping you! Throughout these pages are references to the work of various people with degrees in medicine and/or food science whose findings have helped many people like me and can show you an alternate path to better your health.

All the people and companies who provided supporting information in this book do hold appropriate qualifications and have proved, in their realm of expertise, that their research and recommendations are valid and beneficial to people's health. In the interests of political correctness, you should, where appropriate, be guided by the recommendations of an appropriately qualified health professional person from your home area. But remember, the final test, it's your health at stake here. Just because mainstream health treatment systems are supported and recommended by governments, the wider social results we are seeing for the work of the sickness industry, distinct from the health promotion sector of it, must raise some questions as to where the best results and answers are to be found for an increasing number of us.

You be the final judge. The revelations of this book work for me and can work for you!

THE OBJECTIVE FOR YOU OF THIS BOOK

Getting the best For Your health after health issues

A re you feeling below par, not satisfied with how some or many parts of your health are progressing? Here in this autobiography is the answer, what worked for me, and how you can lift your well-being to a better level of health by applying these same, simple answers for yourself.

If you are one of the many people who, over time, are feeling down and disillusioned by an ongoing mediocre feeling of well-being then here is your answer and guide to help you lift yourself to a better level of health and enjoyment of life.

If you are a long term medication user of any Big Pharma medication and finding you are getting side effects. Check out the listed side effects for that drug & any suggestions they offer.

There is a host of helpful guiding points though this book both for people who are having issues and looking for answers and who are not regular users of prescription drugs. Plus if you are a regular prescribed medication user then there are more answers with natural ways for you to help build your well-being to more desirable levels. Read on!

Prescription medications and their subtle side effects have been a part of my life experience since 2001, when I was fitted with an artificial heart valve. Following that surgery, the constant use of prescribed drugs has for me and can, and does, over time for many users have a real negative effect on my general vitality and sense of well-being because of their acid effect on the body. This low acid effect puts one's body out of balance from our body's ideal acid–alkaline balance. The medical establishment tells us nothing about how to help cope with this affect or even admit it exists.

For the next nine years after 2001, life for me went through this constant rollercoaster of feeling OK at times to awful, from near healthy to flu, depression, lethargy, never properly healthy. If there was some sort of bug going around, it was sure to affect me! I was constantly at a doctor seeking an answer to my unhealthy issues! It has taken *ten years* for me to work out the root causes of my below normal health issues and then apply this learning to dramatically better my health and vitality!

Here's your opportunity to apply this learning to your life over the next *ten weeks* and know what it feels like to be and feel really healthier again!

Live Deliberately; make it your focus to think through your lifestyle and develop and act on a positive plan for your goals in life.

People with diabetic issues may find some helpful insights in this book

MY Aim For this book is For you to Achieve these amazing results For Yourself!

By knowing and understanding the major impact on one's well-being, you are able to do what needs to be done to get your energy and life back—simple, economical, everyday habits and inputs which achieve real results to give you a real lift in your energy and vitality. The answer and solution to improving your health is provided in these pages. Regardless of the particular cause of your 'Oh dear' problem, you will find many things to help you in the following pages.

Stomach gas - wind, acid reflux & diarrhoea can all became the new issues when you pH balance gets too acid. See mid chapter 5 for more on this.

Now is your time to apply all I have learnt. Build your lifestyle around it, seeking the best health and vitality you can for the benefit of your body, mind and soul. The goal here is to provide you with insights from my learning and the learning of many others. Leave those negative experiences of your past life, and get on and start to enjoy your new life. When you feel the benefits and experience of the difference in yourself, you will be inspired to spread the word around your family and friends.

The world we live in is experiencing *massive* change at speeds which, in my youth, were considered inconceivable. We must blend those changes to fit with ways that work best for the benefit of our bodies to ensure we get our desired result of good health for life. It does not fit with nature's way to spend years in declining health before going through more pain in anticipation of a slow, agonising death while during that time being kept alive by the 'sickness industry' but never really feeling and being truly healthy.

We have this amazing body, mind, and soul, the ultimate achievement of evolution and God-given powers in this world. From that base, we now have the ability to take charge and use what nature provides, to enjoy the best nutritional and water supply for our ultimate health benefit. Join with me through these pages and give yourself a better understanding of what options you have and can apply to enhance your health, vitality, and well-being.

Picture below - Me the author August 2013. @ 75 years old.

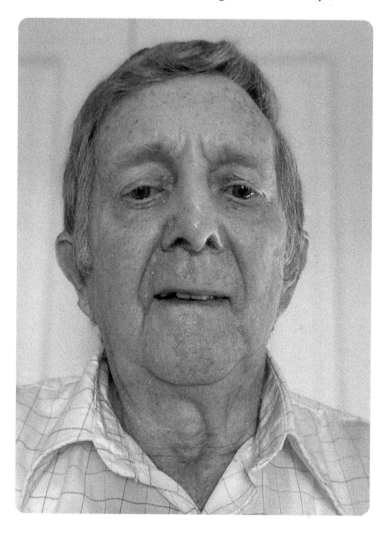

CHAPTER 1

CLAIM YOUR LIFE BACK!

Where Do You Feel You Are on Your Personal Health Scale?

You have had your major health issue diagnosed and either repaired, and/or you are now on a number of medications to help you overcome the negative effects of that trauma to protect you from possible complication effects.

How many different drugs have you been recommended to take?

Have you been provided a full and detailed explanation for likely short- and long-term effects of those chemicals to your body and any likely cross interactions between those chemicals!

What are they designed to do for you?

What benefits do you see and feel?

What negative effects are likely? Some of these you may have to accept as the cost of helping with your major problem. Others may not be revealed to you, but over time, you will find subtle negative effects creeping up in you.

We get prescribed all sorts of medications to help with our health. It's the standard instant fix solution we have been led to believe will solve the problem.

Often, in the short term, the benefits are obvious.

Then over time, you may find yourself not feeling the better health you wanted, or the results fade and you find yourself stumbling from one health issue to another without ever really having any comprehension of what the underlying problem is. Sometimes the real causes of your health issues may be hidden in the combinations of food additives, flavourings, taste enhancers, etc. that are being added to all processed foods and drinks and how these products are reacting to your particular DNA type.

But your health can and will work even better for you *if* you know or work out the answers I provide here!

Otherwise, you may have to stumble along, put up with, and work through a whole list of various effects like I worked through for your answer to better health—if you can figure it out!

How do you feel in relation to your historical healthy normal body?

As the weeks pass, you will normally feel degrees of improvement in your health and well-being. If you simply started taking some drugs on doctor's recommendations, then this change in feeling may be only slight. If you had major surgery and repairs to internal organs, then you will most likely feel a greater lift in your well-being level at first after you get over the trauma of your body repair. Now that's great, but the key point I want to make here is that you need to establish a historical healthy reference point in your mind of when you felt really healthy and vibrant (or a picture of someone you know who is well and healthy). Now having that as your desired benchmark, you can compare how you feel now with that reference point.

Where do you feel you are on the feelings list below?

- dramatically better
- better
- about even/on par
- below desired level
- worse
- simply awful
- simply awful and slowly getting worse.

Where do you fit on that scale?

You will find that by applying the ways of this book, you will automatically work your way up that scale to the 'dramatically better' level. Your health and well-being, both physically and mentally, are your most important assets.

Has the world of New Age surgery and medicine given you this second chance? Now to get the best enjoyment from your renewed life, you can dramatically help yourself by knowing what works from a patient's point of view. It is simply amazing how surgeons have developed ways of maintaining and repairing our bodies so we can have extended life in the same old body. Whether you have had dramatic surgery in your life or are simply on a diet of assorted medications to aid your health, you will find many beneficial insights here.

For you—or someone close to you—taking prescribed drugs at the direction of a medical practitioner's recommendation for the 'benefit' of your (or their) health and well-being is the new way of living. Here it's more about how the drug affects us and how to adjust to living with its side effects, what they are and what you may expect and how you should counter any undesirable effects. The medical establishment either does not know or will not talk about any drugs having subtle side effects as described in this book and mostly choose to ignore you or claim any of these effects as irrelevant.

But there is this one major side effect that is not mentioned, and for some it is only slight. For many of us, it feels more obvious, but we cannot pinpoint what the problem is!

Over time, this effect has a constant 'subtle drag' on your feeling of well-being and energy levels.

Since being recommended to take your prescribed drug, do you find yourself feeling that way?

Feeling not quite 'normal'—the well-being level that you know and feel you should have or that was your norm in earlier life?

Do you find yourself having a whole range of minor negative health experiences?

At each one of these occurrences, you go to your health practitioner and explain the issue, to which he/she responds by prescribing some more medication.

> You then find that more medication tends to not solve the problem—or perhaps it helps with one issue but creates other problems. All that ongoing frustration just adds to that 'dragging' feeling that ails you. You may have had this situation repeating many times since starting warfarin or some other long term medication!

Is this your experience of how and what the world of modern medicine has done and is doing to and for you!

So what is happening here?

What is the problem?

How can you find the solution and answer!

What is the real cause of all these ongoing issues? Perhaps it is time to look outside the box or square!

CHAPTER 2

MY STORY

To give you a perspective on the writer, here's my story so you can perhaps compare your life experience to mine. You may see some or many similar experiences, all of which can give you a lead into why this book will provide real answers and benefits for yourself and those around you. Here you can see that maybe I know a lot on what I'm talking about. After coming through the pain and frustration of this learning experience, I now feel really good that finally life has reached a stage for me where my health and vitality are at optimum levels for my age and life is fun and joyous.

The (Not So) Golden Years of Childhood

Life for me started in the farming country, New South Wales, Australia, back in the late 1940s, on a beautiful section of land which my father built into his dream stud sheep farm. He and my mother were workaholics. Work was the only lifestyle they knew. Having a social life was not part of the weekly plan; more like only once each three months did we spend some time relaxing with relatives or other locals for a few hours. This property had everything to support one's best physical health. As part of the farm workforce along with the sheep, there were horses to ride plus

Kelpie dogs to help work the sheep and cattle. A small herd of milking cows where real fresh full-cream milk was provided for breakfast and to sell. Fresh vegetables in season from the large, well-nurtured vegetable garden. A rose garden and lawns. A mixed-variety orchard of fifty fruit trees. Red and green table grapes. There were egg-laying chickens, turkeys for Thanksgiving and Christmas. Some pigs, plus grain crops to feed them and more. A creek to swim in, in summer and catch fish all year, rabbits, foxes, some kangaroos, and plenty of native bird life, plus the final touch of thirty hives of European bees to pollinate all the plants and provide us with that nectar of the gods—honey. So from that brief description, you can get a good perspective on the concept that I know what I'm talking about when I say I know what real fresh, properly-ripened-before-harvest healthy food does and should taste like, plus how you and your body benefits from living on a good variety of nature's own real food. (More on this in chapters 5 to 9) Despite all that abundance, my parents were stuck in the mindset that there was never enough of anything. So being generous was not normal even though there was actually a substantial amount of wealth being generated by, and flowing through, the family business and home.

The family unit included parents with four children (I was number 3) plus cousins and uncles/aunts on neighbouring farms. Life was very disjointed and emotionally strained, all of which left various emotional scars that have only just been cleared out of my psyche after fifty-plus years. Those events added pressure to my physical health issues. At age nine, I developed serious rheumatic fever (a heart condition), and because of that, I was banned from participating in sport till age fifteen. That left me very much on the outside of school social groups. Another issue adding to my emotional distress! Then three years in boarding school (it felt like a prison camp) during my high school years from age twelve to fifteen was an emotional and social nightmare (particularly because of the total separation from the world of females and hence not learning how to properly relate to them!). After that, I had a year doing a farm management degree at an agricultural college, which I enjoyed. Life from then on went normally until this issue developed in my late 40's

All in My Imagination –
The professionals not Listening/hearing me

As I approached midlife at fifty I began to feel a distinct lack of energy together with a constant and progressive overpowering tiredness. I was spending at least three afternoons a week asleep in addition to seven normal nights asleep. Numerous visits to several doctors gave me no clue to the cause of my condition. Then I had more tests, more doctors and specialists, with still no positive diagnosis to which we could attribute to my lack of energy. Finally, several of these doctors and specialists all decided that my condition was best described as chronic fatigue syndrome, for which they had no recommendations that were of any help to me.

Their final words to me were that I was simply a persistent and repeat whinger for whom they did not have a diagnosis and that I should leave them alone. The message was 'Get over it, get well by yourself, and stop wasting our time and yours!' My feelings at this point, after three years, were of total frustration and disillusion. I felt that these 'experts' really had no defined method to get any insight into my condition. Having spent many sessions with these medical 'professionals', looking for an answer to my poor health, and then having them all infer that it was all basically in my imagination was a real insult! With the aid of hindsight, I realise that a major block for all of them was their total focus on issues relating to their particular specialisation and not one of them looking at the bigger picture of my well-being and other possible causes of the problem. They did not have the holistic approach that I needed.

During all the preceding events, there was one diagnosis that later proved to be a major turning point. A CAT scan revealed an artery aneurysm in my groin. It would require surgery within some years as a safety measure to prevent rupture, I was advised! But this condition was not likely to be a contributing factor in my fatigue issue. More frustration! After being told it was all in my mind, I decided to try the Vegsource cleanse diet, which was a great help. Check them out and connect with the free offers there along the way. Next, I started taking premium nutritional supplements from a relatively new (back then) health sciences company, and the improvement in my health and well-being was amazing over the next few weeks and months. So I thought that was the answer, and to hell with the medical world! So back into the world of work and action, where life was better for a time!

Near-Death Experience

But life is not always that simple! Another year went by with yet another slide in my health. Winter dragged past with almost constant flu symptoms. Then in mid spring, at a meeting with the surgeon who was to repair my aneurysm, the real cause of all my failing health issues was revealed. He had my heart checked before booking me in for surgery. That ultrasound check revealed major leakage of my main heart valve. The aortic valve had more than doubled in size from stretching and was leaking backwards at more than 45 per cent of through flow. Well, no wonder my body was not going as I thought it should. 'It's a wonder you are still alive,' the surgeon said and promptly booked me in for urgent heart surgery within the next week.

Now with the aid of cutting-edge surgery, all was fixed, and an artificial valve replacement was put in my heart. Wonderful! I was fixed and cured, I thought. So there you are—I was saved from the jaws of premature death from poor DNA and body parts by new-world technology. Born again literally in the physical sense!

I give serious thanks to the very capable surgeons who did the work!

Ongoing Prescribed Drugs to maintain my health

The pharmaceutical side of medicine now gets to have its impact on the rest of my life. Several drugs were prescribed for me to take for the remainder of my life as ongoing aids to my health and well-being! The first one I took for a month and then, on reading the side effects list, said, 'No thanks.' The second was a drug designed to reduce the risk of my heart getting too excited or stressed. I took till 2021 when it was changed to a different heart drug after going through an irregular heart beat period which went on for nine months. When having this irregular heart beat issue it dramatically reduces your general energy level by half or more to the point where life seemed that it did not matter if I was alive or DEAD.. This irregular heart beat issue was fixed with electric shock treatment in march 2022 when specialists put my heart beat rhythm back to normal. Thanks again to my persistence and finding a doctor who told me the solution I was looking for. During and after this out of rhythm heart beat issue I also was coping with Stomach gas - wind, acid reflux & diarrhoea. Caused by the new additional drug I had been prescribed after my erratic heart beat issue developed. {this I worked out over subsequent months}. The other drug is warfarin, which started on back in 2001 and still take to thin my blood as a protection from the risk of a clot forming where my artificial heart valve is fitted. A good, valid reason! This taking of warfarin needs the constant checking of one's INR levels to ensure the correct dose is being consumed. As part of this checking process, the daily dose tends to change from time to time as a result of changes in diet habits, seasonal food changes, and a few other variables.

INR (International Normalised Ratio) is an abbreviation that the medical world uses to identify the rating or grading system used to measure your blood's ability to form blood clots. They have developed a preferred reduced clotting ability zone in which they feel it is desirable for the body to operate because of the risk of clots occurring where the artificial heart valve is connected into my heart. Maintaining my blood in this desired INR zone eliminates this risk. Regular tests are done to check where my blood clotting ability fits on this preferred zone and assessments made as to the required amount of warfarin I take to maintain this INR level.

So the saga goes on. While there was a substantial improvement in my health after recovering from the trauma of major heart surgery, my life just did not have the zing to it that I felt it should.

The negative effects of these drugs and the drag on my body still continued. At times, I needed all my energy and determination to get out of this ongoing negative health hole, resulting in this constant 'Oh dear, I don't feel as good as I should and would like to feel.' That was me! The constant irritations and dragging feeling drained my energy, making living just a continuing full-time hard slog. Everything I went to do felt like a major effort that took all my willpower to achieve. That constant 'Oh dear, I just cannot muster the energy to do this' and 'How am I going to get back to the things in life which I once enjoyed doing?'

The major underlying issue here which the medical establishment does not recognise and won't talk about is that your body may be negatively affected by the acidity of some prescribed drugs. This adds to the acid load the body must cope with and helps to put it out of balance, which then makes you feel off! One medical establishment response to this is to suggest you are just depressed and to prescribe further medication! Again, that was a diagnosis given to me. More drugs were prescribed, and more undesirable complications resulted, with no beneficial result! I stoped taking these added drugs after months as there was no benefit to me. The real solution is to understand and recognise that my and perhaps your body is out of balance then act to rectify this imbalance! Your acid– alkaline balance is the real issue. Putting this right is the only answer and a major message of this book!

Fed up with these seemingly regular sickness events interrupting life, I decided to research what I could do to enhance my well-being and get off the treadmill of not quite feeling up to speed. Time for a major change, I thought. My eating, drinking, and lifestyle routine over the past few years had not enabled me to make any real positive change from constantly feeling below my desired optimum health level. I made that insight after reading this book by Neale Donald Walsch, *When*

Everything Changes, Change Everything—very relevant! *That's a great idea!* I thought All the things I had been doing over recent years had not made any real change to my well-being, so 'Time for a change' was the obvious answer. Neale's book is extremely well worded and thought out. His insights are inspiring and help you see things from a different perspective. A great book for support to get you past any crisis in your life or simply help you to see things from a different perspective!

Whilst reading his book, this insight occurred to me: It's my body and the only one I can have this time around, so I am determined to treat it well, do everything I can to get myself back to what I consider full health and vitality should feel like! Applying the age-old quote of 'Let your food be your medicine and your medicine be your food' became the most obvious starting point for me to get a solution for my better well-being.

There it is! It's as simple as that!

A Simple Remedy

Breathe, drink, and eat what nature provides us with in its naturally packaged form, plus plenty of exercise! All work together to lift your energy levels and keep your body in an alkaline state!

The more I researched a healthy way of living, the more proof I got that it is the best and only really effective approach to wellness.

There are a number of things you can do to help yourself with this acid imbalance. It has taken *ten years* for me to work this out, then apply the knowledge and feel it turn into dramatically better health and vitality for me! Here's *your* opportunity to apply *my* learning to your life over the next *ten weeks*!

If you are having ongoing issues with your health, not feeling expected improvements to your well-being, then these insights will enable you to take this new path and give yourself a real lift from the negative effects of some prescribed drugs. This then will enable you to get back in harmony with better health patterns and continue living with health and vitality over the next years of your life.

Learn how to counter negative effects of prescription drugs

The answer to your health issues as recommended by the establishment is to take prescription drugs and continue on that path until told otherwise. While doing this, you often find other issues develop, and the usual recommendation is to add some more drugs. That's fine if it works for you, but there can be developments of subtle side effects that at first seem minor but over time get more complicated. You may even fell better if you simply stop taking the added medicine. Just know the risks if you do this.

The Major Side Effect You Are Not Told

For me—and you may find the same—there was this ongoing merry-go-round of times when, for a while, my health was reasonable and I felt in balance. Then, as sure as night follows day, there would come some interruption to this mediocre state of well-being. On many of these occasions, I would visit my general physician, seeking some help to deal with a health issue. At most of these meetings, the doctor would make a brief assessment of my situation and, most often, prescribe some new medication . . . or more of one that I had had months/years ago. Then they would suggest that this would fix my issue and they would see me healthy within a few weeks. There was never any interest in spending some time to check for contributing issues or if there were other ways to do things that would improve my situation.

Never, ever was there any suggestion made that maybe some of this ongoing variety of medications might actually be part of the problem! This constant up, down, and around, the health merry-go-round, eats at both your physical and mental well-being! Rarely, if ever, until your health gets totally out of control, is any suggestion ever made about what can be done to improve your health. You are left on your own to figure out what better things you can do to support/improve yourself. You must find your own way and use your own initiative to be assured of getting real solutions to help your health.

There is this one perhaps deliberately avoided and neglected side effect of numerous drugs that the mainstream medical and the Big Pharma world do not consider relevant, have not researched, perhaps are not aware of, and hence, do not tell you about.

It is the pH value of the prescribed drugs and their contribution to how your body goes into an unhealthy acidic state. This does, over time, become a very significant factor to your personal level of well-being as you continue the prescribed drug habit. None of the doctors whom I have talked to about this are even aware of this negative effect, let alone interested in encouraging me, the patient, to be aware of it and work to get my body's acid–alkaline balance back to desirable levels for my health benefit. More of this later!

There are a number of things and different approaches you can use to get your body back to an ideal balance on the acid–alkaline scale and give yourself a real lift in energy and vitality. All these approaches enable you to counteract this negative pH effect and get you back to being really healthy. The rest of this book is dedicated to showing you how to do this.

Wow What an insight!

Were the last few pages a major revelation for you? Maybe you want to stop and digest them for a while. What if, by simply changing some long-established patterns of living and adding a few premium nutritional supplements to your diet, you could shift your well-being up some levels? Change up a few gears!

Put your life back into overdrive where you can, will, and do experience the excitement of life's opportunities! Being excited, motivated, and wanting to get fully involved in this incredible journey and experience of *life* . . .

Your doctors have explained the positive effects of your prescribed drugs. Now you can see and know how the negative effects make you feel. Now you have an option to overcome them so that you can live your life with real health and vitality.

By getting your body pH back in balance, you may well find that many of your minor health issues that have developed over the time since you first started using your main prescribed drugs have literally vanished! Just simply cleared up and gone away all by themselves.

The major contributing things that help are:
- the water you drink & it's pH
- your diet
- nutritional supplements
- lifestyle
- your positive/negative thoughts, stress, etc.
- All these will *dramatically* lift your feeling of well-being— in short, show you ways that enable you to move away from that physical and mental state where life is a constant effort to survive and carry on with your daily activities.
- Now that we understand the subtle side effects and the effect they can and do have on your life, let's look at how you can reduce the negative
- effects and improve the quality of your life. The next few chapters deal with specific areas such as food, water, and mindset, and I will detail how you can simply apply better practices to your own life.

Plus do you regularly use a Microwave oven, read about the effects from them we are not told about in chapter Six. This could also be a major part of your feeling bad.

CHAPTER 3

YOUR HEALTH AND VITALITY VERSUS THE INTERESTS OF THE MEDICAL ESTABLISHMENT AND BIG PHARMA

We Live in this New Age world of incredible technical, educational, and social change and development, bringing us unbelievable social and personal convenience and comfort! We have access to a vast array of benefits, most of which we assume are in place first and foremost for the support of our health and well- being. This massive change has brought with it both opportunities and consequences. Few of us have had time or understanding to know how best to cope with and apply these many benefits for our common good. Or perhaps importantly, question any of this advice and 'advances'. Most of us do not even consider that any of the advice given and technological advances developed is anything but good for us! Perhaps it's time to start living deliberately and give serious thought and study to what is really best for our well-being! Move into a new phase of life and leave behind that inclination to react to things based on subconscious conditioning and old animal instinct.

Over the past century, we have seen the random evolution of our food and environment. Large groups with vested interests control much of our western medical, health, and food system. There are also major contradictions in the often devious and manipulative messages given to us as individuals, causing much confusion about what would serve us and our bodies best. These messages are delivered via the media, fast food and supermarket retailers, governments, pharmaceutical companies, and the medical system. What is frightening is the use of all sorts of chemical additives in the processed foods we buy and the drugs prescribed to us by the medical establishment and Big Pharma.

Social responsibility with you, Mr, Mrs, or Miss Citizen, and your best interests comes a lot lower down the list of priorities, *if it exists at all*, within some major corporations. It's not only our minds that are confused! This focus on the taste of food products by adding all sorts of flavour enhancers is another part of the story that has our bodies totally confused too!

There are numerous herbs and spices that all help with taste and digestion and should not be confused with the chemicals mentioned above.

Eliminate the Major Confusion in your Body Response

Do you want the amazing results that your body can deliver if only you listened to what it is really asking for? Your best way to eliminate ongoing confusion in your body is to get your diet in tune with our long-term natural food diet. Avoid all the man-made flavour enhancers, additives, and subtle taste attractions which have proven undesirable effects on our health.

Or would you prefer to be guided by big businesses and those other vested interests that are simply happy to keep information from you that will be in your best interest and sell you their products regardless?

We are now seeing the results of toxic food, water, drugs, and mindset in our society!

This is showing up in wider society as large proportions of the population in first-world western countries develop major health issues.

We do not help ourselves by continuing with our innate desire to live in the same patterns developed throughout our lives, our lack of knowledge and inertia. All slow the change, increase our ill health, accelerate the ageing of our bodies, and bring our death much closer. And it's hard to make changes because the food manufacturers, for example, spend millions researching how to get us hooked. They know exactly how our bodies work and what we crave or what our temptations cannot resist!

The world of cancer research can be seen as a good example of what I am saying here. In fifty years, there has been massive research and budgets spent on cancer research with some benefits here and there. But all during that time and with all the resources thrown at it, little attention has been given to looking at what benefits we could achieve by encouraging the general population to live in a slightly different way— to consume more of nature's real food and thus reduce our risks of the problem to begin with. If you do not ask the right questions, you can be assured of not getting right answers! In fact, all of mainstream western medicine and the pharmaceutical industries are just not interested in any preventative health measures.

Many of us are encouraged to consume an assortment of medications in an effort to help our health with no long-term aim other than the continued consumption of these pills. The world of Big Pharma is the major winner as our bodies struggle to cope with this mix of chemicals that confuses and disorientates our natural healing processes. Big Pharma wants you sick and alive, using their products, not well, healthy, and independent. Definitely not dead! Dead people do not need medicines or use health care!

When some part of your body does not work in its normal healthy way, you get signals and messages via aches, pains, degrees of illness, etc. This is our body's way of telling us that we need to change something in the way we are providing for it. It is simpler and more profitable plus time-effective for the medical establishment and Big Pharma to prescribe you a pill or take some surgical shortcut than to spend the time, plus the physical and mental effort it takes to get you refocused and re-educated on a healthier way of providing for your body.

We are conditioned and preprogrammed through life to expect a quick fix. This, in most cases, does not provide a beneficial long- term solution for your best health. Minimal focus, if any, is placed on encouraging us to eat a diet that works with our body's natural and instinctive expectations.

It's your choice now: either go with what the system encourages and prefers you to eat then live with and suffer the consequences, or choose to live in harmony with nature's preferred diet as detailed through this book and enjoy the benefits for your better health!

What's your decision? Your change to this can be gradual, and you can still enjoy treats. The key point here is to get your major diet balance in ideal proportions based on what nature has designed for us to eat during the next three to six months. You do not need to be a fanatic about your change; simply work toward making the more natural foods the major portion of your diet.

Below is a sample of a common black-box warning on many pain medications. And it's the strongest possible government-ordered warning that the US Food and Drug Administration (FDA) requires on many prescription and over-the-counter medications. This notice of caution appears in the package insert for prescription drugs. And it indicates that the drug carries a significant risk of serious—or even life-threatening— side effects with long-term usage.

The US Food and Drug Administration is warning you to *watch out*. What's more, the FDA even requires warning labels on over-the-counter medications containing common ingredients such as ibuprofen, ketoprofen, or naproxen.

This strong warning is designed to inform consumers about the increased risk of developing the following health issues in their life if they use over-the-counter medications.

- cardiovascular problems
- gastrointestinal bleeding
- heart attack
- kidney disease
- liver failure
- serious skin reactions
- stroke
- ulcers. And more!

On the subject of organic food versus mainstream supplies, much relevant information about percentages or parts per million of undesirable contaminants contained in foods is deliberately left out of published comparisons between organically produced foods and the others.

It means those food products that people go to great lengths to produce pure, clean, healthy, all-natural products with the end aim of enhancing your better health are being deceptively discriminated against when being compared with mainstream commercial production that uses all sorts of chemicals that can, over time, accumulate and have negative effects on us! Many genuine health consultants and specialists highlight this point consistently. We each need to be vigilant and do our homework on this subject then use the knowledge for our best interest!

The Important Question and Its Focus

Ask yourself this:

1. Do you find that the answers you get from your medical advisers give you solutions that make you feel healthier and better after each session you have with them?

2. Is your health and vitality being maintained or continuing to improve after your last health crisis or after the issue was diagnosed and treated?

Your answers here will give you a definite guide for your future course of action to enhance your health!

The quality of the answers we get in life is determined by the quality of the questions we ask. Plus where we look and ask those questions. We don't ask questions just for the sake of it. Let's ask questions which provide answers that cause us to grow, to develop as human beings. Why is it that there are some small communities on this earth who all enjoy good health and vitality into their one hundreds without intervention from our New Age world? And why is it that no one is asking what works in their world and how we can apply that to our own societies? Is this a time to consider a redesign of the way we live? Is it perhaps that we are so settled in our current comfort zone that not enough people want to listen or hear the answers for what really works?

Dr Steven Gundry MD has actually researched the above questions and his findings are very enlightening

CHAPTER 4

THE PH FACTOR

What It Is and Why It Is So Important to Your Well-Being

First, let's get a full understanding of what pH is and what it measures. Put simply, this is our way of measuring the competing forces of *acid* and *alkalinity*. These opposite forces compete in all facets of life at all levels throughout nature. This balance is part of how all nature and life operates.

The really *exciting thing* is to learn about this fact and how you can apply and get great benefit from this knowledge for yourself by using it to enhance your health and vitality. In our body, nature has set the optimum operating pH level at pH 7.4 as the ideal point where most of our body systems operate best. Our body strives to maintain our blood at pH 7.4 at all times and sacrifices all other body function pH levels to maintain that pH 7.4 level of our blood.

Our digestive system and connected parts including pancreas is the one major working system of our body where pH does change down & up as part of normal daily eating, drinking, digestion, food adsorption and waste disposal. When these changing processes of our body are pushed outside body preferred health norms by what we eat and drink, plus new age medications, that is when all the pH issues discussed in this book come into action for worse or better. All the changes in how everything is done over the past 70 years has added to this up & down effect. How you cope with that is what I aim to explain and help you understand. How to live more in tune with adjusting to these changes for your wellbeing.

What we eat and how we live has dramatic effects on that balance, either by helping maintain it at the desired point or forcing it off balance, normally towards the *acid* direction. All alkaline food, alkaline drinks, no medications, positive thought processes, and clean air, when combined, serve to maintain our pH 7.4 ensuring we are able to enjoy fully real health and vitality. The further away from that ideal point our body gets, the more negative the effects on our health and well-being. To measure this effect on yourself, simply measure the pH of your saliva and/or urine. Most 'normal' Western diets lean towards acid then add stress plus the negative pH 6.2 of warfarin, and that's a good indication as to why you are feeling like crap or well below par, because your pH level is most likely way below the optimum level.

Raise and Maintain Your Body pH on a Daily Basis

What we eat and how the body copes with foods from different pH levels has a strong effect on all the variable pH working processes of the body. The major influence here is the actions of our digestive system. This is first primed by chewing our food and mixing saliva with it before swallowing. Then on reaching the stomach, our digestive system produces and adds sodium bicarbonate to the consumed food. This mixes with the food, and a variety of chemical actions take place. The food is broken down into minute-size portions, and its pH is raised to over 8, ready for the journey through the small intestine. A by-product of our digestion process comes from the 'baking soda' that sometimes reacts with water to produce hydrochloric acid. This, being a heavier chemical, falls into the stomach's inbuilt collection zone, called the gastric pits, as part of the natural sorting action designed by our body before the food gets to our small intestine. (Refer to the explanation three paragraphs down on busting the established digestive myth.)

After all this sorting, the raised pH food mixture from the stomach then moves into and through our small intestine, where our blood gets in close contact with the whole mix and allows for good interaction on near-equal pH terms between our blood and the small intestine contents, where food absorption happens. There, each individual blood cell chooses whatever particular compounds it needs to then transport it around our body to feed or store in our body.

When the body's pH level is under stress, our stomach's ability to perform the complex and interconnected processes required does not work properly, which then results in a whole range of follow-on negative effects throughout the body! These effects can show up under all sorts of labels or names given them by the old-world medical establishments and sickness industry. That industry makes no attempt to relate any of those effects to your body pH level.

In most instances, finding the solution to it by getting your pH back on track would be the simplest and best answer to most of the health issues you have. This is your way to easily and simply put your health totally in balance and on track. Get your pH right, and everything else goes right for you the way nature designed it and intends it to work for your optimum health and vitality!

Busting the Established Digestive Myth

Our established understanding of how the stomach works has never seemed quite right to me, and on researching this book, the real answer has provided the proof of that.

The idea that our food and digestive system pH has to gyrate down the pH scale as it leaves our mouth into the stomach where it is surrounded in a strong acid solution during the pre-absorption process and then magically gets transformed back up the pH scale as it moves from our stomach into small intestine where absorption of useful food parts by our blood without negative effects does not fit with reality. Can you imagine your body being able to change the pH level of all your food down the scale by three to four big points then keep it there and protect your stomach lining from all that acid while digestion occurs? And it also has some inbuilt measuring switch to inform the stomach that its digestion job is finished and the next step to clear away the acid. Then it proceeds to reverse the pH process and drive all that food back up the pH scale by four to six points with the end objective point being pH 8.4 for the food to be ready to travel into your small intestine.

Science does not allow the changing of pH levels so dramatically without major energy inputs, side effects, and by-product results! We do not have any indicators that conclusively show this process actually occurs in the body. Here is my understanding from various sources of what really happens and how nature has produced a system that short- circuits and avoids most of the requirements of the previous paragraphs. View the pH scale chart near the middle of this chapter to get the picture!

The Current Digestive Theory

It turns out that the old myth of strong acid pH stomach is simply a by-product of the interaction between the food and the sodium bicarbonate that our body produces and mixes with the food for digestion. This then forms some hydrochloric acid as a by-product of the digestion process. The acid falls into the gastric pits of the stomach where it collects for disposal via our urine. (Older studies have found this acid and made the assumption that the stomach uses a strong acid process because of that discovery. Many choose to blindly hold fast to the 'strong acid work done in the stomach' point of view, even though it defies the logic presented in the previous two paragraphs.)

Our body collects these atoms of acid and disposes of them via our urine. As this process has gone on, most of the stomach contents have actually been raised in pH by the sodium bicarbonate produced in our stomach as the interaction with the food goes on. (Is that why they call it baking soda? Because it helps things evolve?) This one-way journey on the pH scale only requires one or two points' climb for most alkaline foods.

The bigger move up the pH scale for strong acid foods is the reason we feel heavy and drained after eating large portions of acidic foods. Our stomach's digestive process has had to be cranked up to deal with the strong acidic foods, and our body then must deal with clearing out the extra acid to get rebalanced. This must be done before the food moves through our small intestine. All your body's energy sources rally to cope with the process. Added to that heavy feeling is the extra time it takes for our stomach to make all those adjustments happen. That's why lions always lie down for a rest after having a substantial meal. It gives their body the time it needs for digestion to work. By staying with lighter alkaline foods, we avoid all that discomfort and wasted time, especially if you are one who enjoys action more than sleeping! If you prefer the more acidic foods, then test the level in your urine and learn where you are on the pH scale.

The proportions of alkaline versus acid foods that we consume have a very direct effect on where our body systems measure on that scale. Also note that as your pH level drifts towards acid, it takes a proportionately bigger input of pH alkaline foods and water to counteract the acid effect. Up to ten times as much pH alkaline intake can be required to get you back to the ideal balance point of pH 7.4.

Your intake of a regular dose of low pH medicine adds another load to this imbalance factor. Over time, this subtle drag builds and compounds to the point where all sorts of health issues can become more of a problem for you. Our standard modern-day western diet can, for many, be a contributing factor in this downwards drag on our body pH level.

Test Your pH and See for Yourself

Measuring your saliva and urine pH levels is a quick, simple, and easy two-minute exercise best done first thing in the morning before drinking or eating to be sure of getting an accurate result! For most people on the typical western diet, this test will give a result of between pH 6.5 and 7.0 for your saliva. Your urine test may give a slightly lower reading than your saliva, but as long as it's above pH 6.5, you are probably in reasonable condition. For me, it was a real shock to get readings of pH 6 for saliva and pH 5.8 for my urine on my first test. No wonder I was not happy with my state of well-being!

Most health food shops will have a test kit you can purchase. Be sure to buy a kit that only measures the middle section of the pH scale. From 5.5 to 8 is the most informative test for accurate and precise test results.

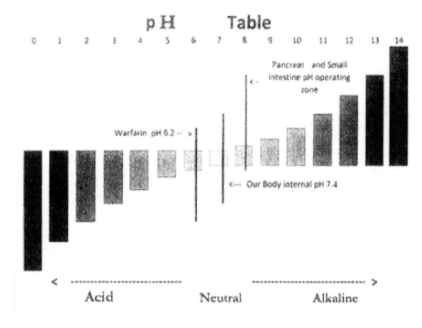

These are some of the pH measures that our body works to Body internal / blood near pH 7.4

Small intestine & Pancreas pH 8

Warfarin pH 6.2

As our saliva and urine pH gets below pH 7, the negative effects start to become evident, becoming even more so under pH 6.5 as our ability to maintain optimum health is reduced and we become susceptible to the invasion of a whole range of negative health issues. From the above you can see that Warfarin is below many of our body's preferred pH levels & hence the issues exposed in this book. to see a visual Look at what I'm saying here see the pH scale chart

It is also important to be aware that the change in degree of strength along each point on the scale works in the logarithmic progression way. That means the change from 7 to 6 provides a concentration factor change of 10. Then the second big point change along the scale from 6 to 5 provides a concentration amplified change factor of 100. The third big-point move along the scale provides a concentration amplified change factor of 1,000. Each extra point along the scale continuing to increase in strength tenfold from the previous until we get to zero which is car battery acid strength! The same is true as you go up the alkaline side from 7, but this rarely happens to anyone! The vital point to understand here is that once your pH readings get any more than 0.8 to 1 big point away from the ideal at pH 7.4, then this amplified strength factor really starts to bite and, hence, dramatically increases one's feeling of being off balance and unwell. The scale above is drawn to provide a visual insight into the degrees of change to the pH concept and the importance of you keeping your body near the desired balance point.

Getting Your pH Right Will Dramatically Improve Your Health and Vitality

Having your body pH as close to, or into, the alkaline side of the pH scale is the most important message you can learn and apply from this book. For me, the transformation from low energy and feeling negative to feeling healthier, motivated, energised, and inspired has been truly amazing.

I do have relapses at times, but the general lift has changed my life for the better in a *big* way. In a matter of weeks, my personal pH urine and saliva readings went up from pH 5.8 to pH 7, and the benefits this has brought to my health and well-being continue to amaze and inspire me. As part of this process of change, you may need to consider and change how you think and view the world from the mental perspective to achieve the full benefit from all this. Remember, thoughts manifest into things; what you think and focus on is what you become and what you get from life. Look in the mirror of your life to see the results. More on that later, in chapter 10, about living deliberately, reducing worry and stress, and your attitude to—and working with—the available magic of your mind. The degree of change needed for you to benefit from this pH effect may be relatively minimal depending on your DNA strength but it works, thats my point.

Your Body pH Level and Your INR Reading

Warfarin users, please note there is minimal relationship between your pH levels and likely readings of your blood INR. You can have saliva and urine tests results of around pH 6 or saliva and urine tests of pH 7.5. Regardless of your pH test result, your INR level test will reveal a constant and consistent result of your blood's clotting ability. Therefore, all warfarin users can feel secure in the knowledge that by moving the body's pH levels towards more alkaline, the only change you will have is one of improved well-being, feeling better, healthier, and more energised. Your blood INR remains unaffected by any changes in body pH readings.

You can buy a pH test kit from here. www.easyph.com. au Or find one at your local swimming pool shop. The protein figures are from other sources. There may be some cases where perhaps some entries could be better placed, but the important point here is the overall message of this book, which is a diet based on natural, unprocessed, fresh, raw (where appropriate) foods that achieve good health.

In the book *The pH Miracle* by Robert O. Young, PhD, and Shelley Redford Young, there is a full explanation as to why and how this pH factor works for us. If you are one who likes to know the full facts and research behind the story, then be sure to get the latest *revised and updated* edition of their book. The reinforcement provided as to why this works is truly inspiring.

A less technical book, which expands and explains many of the same concepts, is *The pH Balanced Diet* by Bharti Vyas and Suzanne Le Quesne.

Living in the Optimum pH Range

What these people share and have in common with other authors, referred to in chapter 4, is fundamental to my overall message here. The importance of having your pH level in the optimum range is the *key* factor that you need to comprehend from this book.

Having your saliva pH level at 6.6 to 7.4 can provides a whole range of health benefits for you, all of which come totally naturally. No effort, no stress, no secret formula! Just go with the flow and drink, eat, and live in tune with the products of the sun, soil, and water. It's simply the way nature designed your body to perform best.

Maintaining your body at this desired pH level becomes second nature when you get into the routine of high-quality pH+ water combined with premium fresh vegetables and fruits served as nature presents them, without additives. Your natural resistance to disease and infection works better, which flows on to you being healthy all the time. No interruptions from the world of bugs and diseases. Simply enjoy being healthy!

There is a whole host of people who have cured themselves from a variety of degenerative diseases by changing to living this way. They are quoted in the books recommended in this book, and further links to testimonials are also included. My own findings of being much more resistant to all those common ailments and diseases, which are constantly annoying for most of us, is for me the front-line reinforcement of the fact that this is the answer to the good health that you are looking for!

On the negative side of this pH balance, the further down the scale into acid territory your body is, the more health issues you will be bothered by and forced to cope with. Many more stresses just seem to appear in your life, thus making your whole life much more difficult and frustrating!

You might want to read that paragraph again to get the full point of what it says.

We really are at a crossroad here

The decline in general health of a big portion of western society and the strain on healthcare is real reinforcement that we are at a crossroads. Please be reminded that I, the writer grew up on a mainly cooked and substantially carnivore diet. So to choose to make this change has been a major shift for me, but the health benefits dramatically outweigh any desire to stay with old patterns and habits.

So why is a diet based on vegetables and fruit, mainly raw, so good?

The fibre in raw, unprocessed food acts as a broom to keep your intestinal and colon walls clean, thus enhancing your digestive processes. When food is cooked, the intense heat destroys its life. As this cooked food goes through your stomach, the cleaning effect is diminished and some particles stick to your intestinal walls. Over time, this coating builds and putrefies resulting in all sorts of toxic effects plus clogged intestines and colon. Cooked foods do sustain life, but they *do not* have the power and enzymes that allow your body's atoms and cells to regenerate, rebuild, and properly repair/sustain your life forces. Hence the continued consumption of all cooked food simply speeds the degeneration process of your cells and tissues. Also allowing, over time, the development of all sorts of health issues and body part failures!

With that insight, you are better able to understand the essential reason you need to consume a substantial part of your diet as raw food. By doing this, you are giving yourself and your body the life-force nourishment with which your cells and tissues can thrive, the way nature designed you to work best, thus providing your body with nature's best energy forms and all its strongest building blocks to support and repair your health. By going down this path, your body can, and will, heal itself, plus you will not need all these New Age medications & health food supplements to block pain messages and generally confuse your body. As you work through this process of getting your food sourcing and diet on track, it is equally important to spend some time and mental exercise on reinforcing your positive mental attitude and outlook. More of this in chapter eleven.

You may find that the increased consumption of raw vegetables actually increases the amount of warfarin that you need to take. That's fine. The important point to be focusing on here is *you*, feeling better. Your body is better able to deal with the extra warfarin because of your better energy levels.

A Word of Warning -re strong alkaline water

It is possible to overdo alkalinity.

These are some of the symptoms you may experience if you are over the 7.5 pH level on your saliva and urine tests:

- irritation and discomfort in the eyes, swollen tear ducts
- hand tremors, involuntary muscle twitching, and sensations of numbness or tingling in the face, arms, or legs
- nausea and vomiting
- light-headedness
- confusion.

If you feel the above symptoms or other unusual issues bothering you, simply reduce your alkaline intake or add more acid foods and drinks to your immediate food and drink intake till the symptoms subside. If the symptoms do not abate after letting your pH go lower, then you should look for some totally different cause to your undesirable symptoms.

Hopefully this chapter has explained the importance of achieving and maintaining the right levels of alkalinity in your body and the great benefits that can be yours for the taking! Read on to learn how you can further alkalise your body

CHAPTER 5

YOUR BODY'S CRY FOR WATER

The major component of our body is water. So it makes total sense to give your body the best available. Society and the mainstream medical world today have totally ignored this fact. In fact, they actually add to the degrading of our daily drinking water by adding chlorine, fluoride, and a few other chemicals, all for the benefit of protecting our health. It is better than contaminated water, but you get best results from really clean, pure, energised water! Only a small minority of medical professionals make this very important point that really pure water is your best choice! For you to have the best performance from your body, this is your only choice! In its natural and most energised form, pure water is what you must drink for optimum body and mind function.

Why Excellent-Quality Water is a Must

The number-one priority is the purity and energy of the water you drink. The current accepted idea is that the body is 70 per cent water. Muscles are 75 per cent water. Vital organs average around 90 per cent water; blood, 94 per cent water. But you should add to those percentages allowance for the fact that all our body building blocks of proteins, cells and body parts contain a substantial portion of inbuilt water. Science is still learning how important water structures are to our body make-up. Dr Gerald Pollack, senior research professor at the University of Washington, USA, is a leader in this field of learning. Listen to his talks with Dr Joseph Mercola on YouTube for more on this subject or read his books.

Consuming low-energy water results in a whole host of poor energy throughout the body and results in a substantial drop in your ability to enjoy life, Clean, pure energised water is your only healthy option!

What are all the foreign bodies and toxins in your water supply doing to your kidneys and body?

Since getting into this whole new health-conscious routine, I have been using a four-stage water filter to clean my drinking water that comes out of the government supply here where I live. To reinforce the point of how much garbage is contained in my local supply and yours is probably similar!

We are constantly being told that our hydration levels are out of balance. Drinking pure pH-positive energised water is the most effective and simplest way to restore that balance. The speed at which you rehydrate and lift energy levels will absolutely amaze you when you consume pH-positive water! Try it for yourself, and feel the results! Look at the drawn image and photograph of snowflake crystals to give you the full picture and insight into what water does in building complex systems and patterns. Also be aware that if the water has a negative energy load it will NOT freeze into the beautiful patterns you see on U tube

Have a look here for some pictures of snow flake crystals. Log into www. youtube.com then open this video page list on the youtube search bar. masaru emoto water experiment or Wilson Bentley

Back in the 18th century Wilson Bentley did a whole lot of research and book writing on this subject. You can also find some of his work on YouTube. You may have to register or sign into Youtube to get access to the detail pictures for this subject. Below are two sample images to give a small indication of the complexity that water can develop.

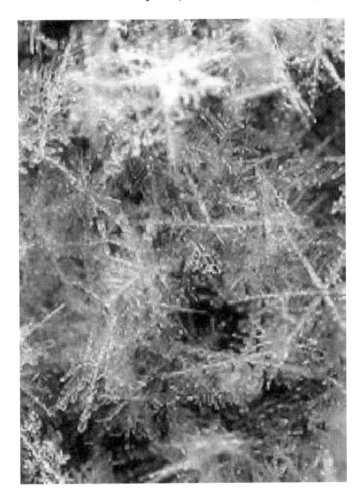

Here above and below are two sample pictures as examples of the complexity into which water freezes.

There are thousands of variations into which snow forms from water! You can see on those web pages This same innate desire to develop into complex patterns and systems is a vital part of the natural process which water undertakes to build all the complex workings in our body.

Water has natural surface tension, which you can see when you place a few drops on a flat surface. It can be seen by the way the edge of the water tends to naturally round itself and resist spreading thinly across the surface. This surface tension factor directly relates to how well all the fluids flow through your body and around your body cells. Water has an energy memory as described by *Masaru Emoto*, later in this chapter.

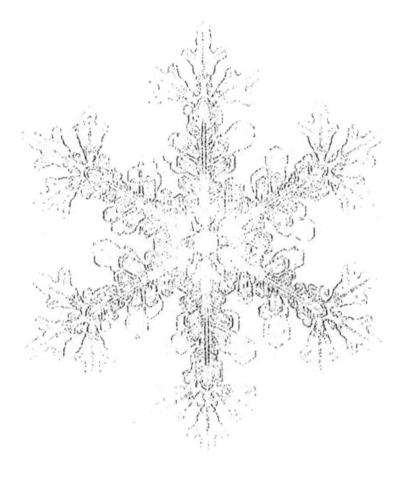

Effects of negative energy on water

If you apply negative and microwave energy to water it will NOT freeze into the snow flake patterns. The negative energy effect destroys the natures natural memory built into water. More on that by *Masaru Emoto.* Getting the energy right in the water you drink is important. That's what the "Bole bungsplatte energy board" below does for you. Water with higher pH and positive vibration has lower surface tension; this gives a dramatic and dynamic lift to all your body fluid circulation systems!

Your blood circulates better and more effectively. Your body's nerve communication system connects faster and more effectively as the cell-to-cell connections are enhanced by this free flow of softer water in your body. There is an amazing degree of inbuilt energy and connectivity in water. The ideal example of this is to look at the vast variety of formations and shapes into which water builds itself as snowflakes develop. It's as if there is an intuitive desire in every molecule of water to build special magic into its and our world. You will, and can, feel the difference within minutes, the first time you have a drink of energised water.

Enhance your vitality and well-being by working with this available energy store. Energised water enhances a whole network of marvellous connections and conduction work in your body! Water has its own inbuilt desire to build into varied and complex patterns, all of which are part of a grand design plan. Applying positive energy, love, and tender care to your food, water, and yourself all adds to this; plus giving thanks as you live is the final blessing.

Going back to my snowflake example, on the higher-consciousness level, research has shown and proved that if you apply positive thoughts like 'This water is blessed with love,' as snowflakes develop, you can have an impact on the results like the picture illustrated above. Alternatively, if you focus negative energy on the snowflake during development, then the result is a mishmash of broken and badly formed patterns or none at all. Applying positive or negative energy can have similar effects in your body. Putting good energy into your body in terms of positive thinking, food, and drink provides good results! As you do this, your whole being becomes more in harmony and produces real positive results in all facets of your life. Working with this positive process of thought and nutrition will, and does, enhance your vitality and well-being at all levels.

The dictionary describes *harmony* as Agreement in action, opinion or feeling.

The way parts combine well together or into a whole to achieve a positive result.

In music, an agreeable combination of notes sounded simultaneously.

All the great religions and, more recently, science have proved this. Look at the research sources below for support and validation on this.

NASA has researched this.

The German Aerospace Institute in Stuttgart has researched this.

Dr Masaru Emote from Japan has done massive research on how positive and negative energy affects water, all of which can be directly related to how and why you react to positive and negative energy in your life!

The Bible talks about this and recommends we should bless our food and water!

Water responds to positive energy from inspired music.

Water has memory similar to how a plastic disc has memory of a movie—just like your DVDs.

There is a vast store of supporting information about this subject available. Research the subject for yourself on YouTube. Search for Masaru Emoto, or Water Memory.—there is a whole host of presentations which reinforce and prove this point. The information sources are all noted on these presentations. What you see and learn will absolutely amaze you. It also reinforces why we should bless our food and water before eating and drinking. A fundamentally important point when doing this is to tune into our alpha and theta brainwave state when and while doing this blessing to ensure our proper real connection with our higher consciousness to give the best results! Check this out and see the results. Positive energy into your body gives you positive health results!

Modern day science / medicine and the big biz food world refuse to accept that any of this subtle energy effect on water can show up in our bodies as health issues and other negative effects so therefore refuse to talk about it.

The first step for me in this journey of discovery about water was to stop drinking local supply tap water, which contains a mixture of chlorine and other chemicals, all of which have negative effects on our bodies! Plus it can have a pH level lower than what best suits your better wellbeing. After spending only a few months drinking mostly bottled spring water I was able to notice an improvement in energy level and generally felt better.

Before writing this book back in 2012 and having been through the learning process of what works better, re water pH I came across a new to the market water filter which had an inbuilt magnetic pH raising mechanism.

After getting this new pH raising filter I was able to cease spending money on bottled spring water and got better results for my continued better health & well being. Unknown to me the working life expectancy of this magnetic pH raising device and filter was only about 6 to 8 years.

As we moved into the 2020 years and not knowing that this magnetic pH modifier was failing me. I began to notice a deterioration in my health, and did not relate it to the failed pH modifier. You must question /check everything when things are not going as expected! There were other irregular heartbeat issues also affecting me during that period which tended to hide the point that it was mostly my poor water intake causing these issues.

Stomach gas - wind, acid reflux & diarrhoea

Stomach gas - wind, occurred quite often in afternoons & evenings, acid reflux & diarrhoea all became the new issues which would seriously interrupt my well being for the next 2 years while I tried to diagnose the cause and answer. The diarrhoea in varying degrees went on for the whole 2 years +. The cause of the diarrhoea in me may well be my using my microwave oven far too much as detailed under that heading in the next chapter. On occasional days my evening and nights would be ruined by a reflux event at monthly to several weeks occurrences during 2021 & 2022. It seemed to be caused by a mix of some modest amount snack foods like potato crisps and beer, ginger beer or low pH water, or some other main evening meal that had a high salt / acid content. This then would totally block progression of my digestion process. The end result being the vomiting of all food & drink that I had consumed after about 5 pm that day. The worst of these occurrences happened in the evening after drinking water with crisps on the completion of the installation of a new multi filter with a Carbon filter & bypass waste as the final stage in January of 2023.

That filter dramatically lower's the water pH; un known to me at that time. And hence caused me a major reflux / vomiting event that lasted till the short hours of the morning. The medical establishment general practitioners had few workable solutions to offer but gave me prescription's for pills that suppress or hide the problem which I found at full strength dose just made the issue worse for me., It was suggested to me that my issue was poor workings of the throat valve where it connects to my stomach and this cause irritations and the reflux.

When I checked the pH of the carbon filter water from the new device I had just installed, it was obvious that low pH water had been annoying me randomly for the past 2 years! Getting the pH changing water ionizer described below has been a major fix for stomach & reflux issues for me. Amazing! and my learnings about Microwave ovens & why you should not use them on any regular basis.

Get a pH changing water ionizer

After that insight came a real lift, when I added a new device that not only filters the water but also raises the pH to the more desirable 7+ pH range of your choice. I found it best to use the lower pH+ setting so as to have water just above the pH centre ranges.

The "Vevor water ionizer" Sold by a mail order company called **Vevor**, with branches in USA, ENG & AUST. The settings are variable and you can set it to suit what works best for the change required to your mains supply in coming water. This device uses a small amount electricity from your mains supply to change the water pH as it passes between energised plates inside the device. A real major winner and probably available from various suppliers in different countries.

Having had more time using pH raised water of different levels as per the meter on the Vevor device. I have found that the best level to use from my experience is 7.5 pH water. You may have to mix the vevor output of "Filtered water and Alkaline one" to get that result; pH above that may tend to give you alkaline side effects listed under sub heading "A word of warning" at the end of chapter Five.

Are you constantly troubled by "acid reflux" tummy issues by causes unknown or other long term medications; then you best start using a Vevor water ionizer now. The standard start setting is "Alkaline Two" setting for your daily drinking water. But you will need to work out for yourself what alkaline water level best suits your body. Use the end of chapter 4 as your guide to what suits you, below alkaline 8 may be better. When you make this change you will find all your reflux issues just stop happening and you can stop using all those other chemist products to suppress the problem.! Over the next weeks - months you should keep in mind the alkaline effects warnings and adjust the alkaline level of your water intake to balance your wellbeing while eliminating your reflux issues.

Comparable devices and also ones that work by magnetic influence & no electricity, by other manufacturers may be available with or without variable pH settings, but this one is what I found.

This change back up to my desired well being state over the next few weeks has been quite AMAZING and uplifting! This Vevor filter requires it's own supply tap. it comes with a tap system and hoses you can connect to your main sink water spout but I found it better to either connect it to your seperate drink water tap on your sink or put the whole device in your laundry and use a T junction to connect off your wash machine cold supply. This eliminates the risk of running hot water through it by accident. Plus no hoses or electric wires around your sink and you can simply do a once a day or less often session to get your pH modified water & turn off it's power when done. If you have an existing filtered drink water tap you can connect to that and get the benefit of more filters reducing the filter load on the Vevor.

In addition to the above I have been using a "Bole bungsplatte energy board". from grander as per below since 2012. This clears all the negative energy out of the water that may develop during the filtering and pH changing processes

The Grander water filter System

Grander supply a water calming board they call "Bole bungsplatte energy board". that has great calming effects on treated water as described earlier in this chapter. A real PLUS for your better water intake and health!

From a different perspective the Grander Company have developed a system which is a onetime only or one off purchase. Their system produces healthy energised water without moving parts or consumable components to wear out or that need replacing. Thus giving you the benefit of an economical and permanent environmentally friendly solution, which can be used with all types of water without using on-going additives.

The water energising device which you can buy from GRANDER energises water as you store it, or pass your water supply through it. You can fit a permanent 'Grander' system in your home and have all the benefits and eliminate the ongoing cost of buying water. The hydration properties of this water are amazing; the company recommends a holistic approach to hydration with the focus on not how much you drink, but how much you absorb. Often people are encouraged to drink large volumes of water per day by health practitioners to correct dehydration, with little benefit as the water they are drinking is simply not absorbable.

You will have heard the saying: "When the fish are sick, change the water".

Have a close and serious look at what you are currently drinking. Compare it's purity to what Nature could provide a century ago. Is it the best for your health and vitality? You may well find yourself being quite shocked if you are using what comes through your kitchen tap. When you make the change you will taste the difference and feel it all through your body and wellbeing.

CHAPTER 6

YOUR FOOD

Old and new Habits Holding Back your Health

We have all become very accustomed to a routine of selecting a mix of foods and go through the intensive process to prepare them for cooking, boiling in water, roasting, steaming, or boiling in oil as our routine meal preparation process. Or the easy & more expensive option - get your meal as a take away.

Microwave Ovens –
What we are not told & what you should know.

Do you use a microwave oven, we are told they are a great convenience aid for our kitchens and fast life style. BUT did you know they were banned in the USSR in the 1980's. Here are more insights as to why they are so bad for your health and long term wellbeing from notes I found on these two web sites. Steptohealth.com & Medicaldaily.com microwave's safety. They go on to list negative affects that should scare you, plus all of which I am reluctant to expand on here due to USA censorship suppression of the subject years ago.

Nature does not use microwave energy for any of it's powering of natures plants and animals.

The use of microwave energy for heating our food is totally a new age man made idea and way of doing things to provide so called convenience time savers with no regard or serious study into their possible long term negative affects.

The madness of big biz, health and politics allowing vested interests to control our lives in ways that only benefit their profit numbers. The short answer re you and microwave ovens, is you are best to simply leave it as a decoration in your kitchen, but NEVER use it or leave it in the shop.

After looking at the web sites suggested above you can find more on Google.

For more reinforcement on this negative point about microwave heating effects to see it for yourself using this study using 2 or more plants. One to water with Microwaved water only & the other with regular tap water. Boil some water daily in your microwave oven and let it cool & be careful not to open the microwave oven for a minute or two after it stops as there are risks involved talked about on those web sites re boiling water in microwave ovens. Then water pot plants which gets plenty of sun but no rain daily with that water. What you will see happen over the next few weeks / months will reinforce my point here! Water the other plant with tap water that has been boiled on a conventional stove & then cooled.

I have done this test for my self on leafy lettuce plants over a five week time. The first two weeks showed minimal change but from then on the microwave watered plant showed real signs of negative health issues. I would choose not to eat it. As that is the affect of microwaved water on a plant. Microwaved food or water affects on your body will be undesirable or worse. Why risk these negative affects on your digestive system & general wellbeing!

You can see some videos of this on YouTube. Open the YouTube web site and type "microwave water on plants" into the YouTube search bar, Plus there are other talks about microwave oven issues there as well.

For most of us, little consideration is given to the positive and/or negative affects on our body of this established food preparation routine. It's what our parents did, and we simply continued the same old pattern.

Any affects on us and or body tend to be subtle and get worse very slowly over many months and years, the vast number of people with serious health issues in our time should reinforce your concerns! If you only warm your coffee once a week you may not notice any affect but the more you use a microwave the more your body will react to the negative affects and the more likely you are to notice undesirable changes in your wellbeing. If you defrost/warm/cook one meal a day this warning will certainly apply to you.

Over the past few years I got lazy and was eating pre-packed prepared meals from the supermarket which all have heating instructions for using either conventional oven or Microwave. I noticed these negative affects on me, general aches all over at times, Diarrhoea that would not go away, possibly even the early stages of leaky gut syndrome as my intestine was subject to the negative energy affects from Microwaved food.

At the start of 2023 year, I became aware of this microwave oven issue and stopped using it, since then all the bad feelings and issues have substantially reduced to totally gone away.

In the old world several generations ago people seemed to have less health issues. Maybe it's another reason why so many new age people have health issues.

Food absorbs energy much like water does as described back in chapter 6 by *Masaru Emoto*. Your stomach may not recognise and therefore does not absorb negatively energised food/water. That's why the above issues develop in food which contains water as it's major component.

If you have been buying packaged prepared meals that are frozen, organise your self and give the pack time to thaw out before you put in your conventional oven in an oven proof dish . The pack may have microwave heating instructions on it but you best simply ignore them for all the above reasons and your better ongoing health. You can look up a few examples of the effects of microwaved water on plants on youtube. Here's one I found, the affected plant grew smaller with smaller leaves & less flowers. some dead leaves & flowers over 2 months. Log into www. youtube.com then open this video page list on the youtube search bar. microwave water on plants

These effects may only seem mild and slow to show but if it's you and you are having other health issues it all helps to slow you down / make you sicker. The world of science has not made any serious attempts to diss-prove these negative claims about microwaves and the traditional doctors of medicine just will not go there. Your body will tell you the answer.

Whats good for you & your food preparation ways

Old habits get very firmly entrenched as the way to do things. As an integral part of this complex preparation and cooking routine, we are constantly shown how adding all sorts of sauces and shortcut taste enhancers make this process produce a better, tastier result. Plus we have that desire for the taste of cooked meat and/or fish to make the whole dining experience more inspiring and to end in giving you that full feeling.

Add to the above the traditional perceptions that whoever is preparing the meal has not done their job unless they have spent and been seen to spend a substantial time organising and preparing the meal. After years of spending that time, people develop the mindset that spending time is a very important part of the food preparation process for them.

How would you respond to a situation where preparation and serving is shorter and simpler, where you then have the opportunity to spend that time on other things? You may feel threatened! You may find this variation in routine quite confusing or demanding at first. Or you could find yourself actually enjoying the change! Work through these feelings, and as your body responds to the changed diet, you will feel rewarded for the determination you have applied to make the change.

This feeling of fullness after eating is, again, what we have been conditioned to. But in fact it is the signal from your stomach that the hard work of digesting this mix of foods has now to be given full priority by your body. All your available energy is taken from your other bodily functions to deal with the increased need of your stomach to deal with this 'usually more than you need' serving. Also, the different foods— for example, protein and carbs—would digest better if eaten at separate times and thus allowing your body to use less energy to process the vegetables and lighter foods on their own. Plus you would gain the added nutritional benefit from the vegetables when they are cooked less!

When you are eating poorer quality food, this feeling will be achieved after much bigger quantities are eaten, leading to an uncomfortable feeling of fullness. This is followed by a lack of energy as your body is coping with the huge quantity consumed and using all its resources to digest the oversized serving. Obviously over time, this leads to weight gain and obesity, then sickness such as heart disease, cancer, and diabetes.

There is a totally different sort of feeling or awareness that comes into play when you have eaten sufficiently to satisfy your nutritional needs, which is well worth the experimentation to experience! This happens when you have had a small meal of nutritionally sound, properly ripe fruits and vegetables. You find your taste buds telling you this is really good food! Your stomach very soon tells you also that this is really good food as it comprehends the complete nutritional value in what you have just had. Then you are very aware that yes, you are fed and satisfied.

Enhance This Process by Juicing

This nutritionally satisfied feeling builds even quicker and stronger when you first put your selection of raw vegetables and/or fruit through a juice-extracting machine and then drink the juice as soon as it is made. By doing this, you bypass the body's need for your stomach to do all the hard work, breaking down the food particles ready for absorption. It is useful to get into the habit of 'chewing' the juice; this adds saliva to the mix as you consume it. This helps speed the digestion process. Your body can get straight to absorbing the nutrients and feel a very quick and sustained energy lift without feeling full. Consider the time taken and the cost of the juicer as an investment in your better health. The pay-off is very rewarding. You may be surprised!

Use only fully ripe and organically grown foods to achieve the above benefits. It may take some time for you to source a selection of properly developed foods. You may even be driven to grow the produce yourself or find someone who does and arrange to share some of theirs! The major reward here is that when you experience this result, you get to know and feel the full pleasure and total understanding, at all levels, of the message your body is giving you. Listen to your body, and be sure when this event occurs to savour it, and reinforce the importance of this message in your mind and body. Well done! This is that special point when full understanding of our special connection with true healthy nature flows through to us. From now on, you know very decisively what works best and what course to pursue.

Wow! Was that a totally new way of describing and understanding your body's messages, telling you the *truth* about good holistic food?

On the other hand, opposing this insight is that a large proportion of processed food today has a vast assortment of taste- and flavour-enhancing products and chemicals combined within. All these designer chemicals are made to deliberately confuse your senses so you think you are getting normal, natural, real food when, in fact, a lot—maybe even all of them—are there simply to entice you to eat that particular product in increasing amounts! Your body and your degree of wellness are your best gauges.

Detoxing

Do you feel and look in tune with nature's design, or are you out of balance? If you feel out of balance, maybe you need to detox and have your senses properly tuned in so you notice these differences. It may take some time for you to detox your system at first and be sure to take care and detox properly (and maybe slowly). It can be dangerous to flood the body with toxins that have been stored in your cells if the body can't quickly and adequately eliminate them.

It is in your best interest to consult a professional who can walk you through the process of cleansing and detoxing safely. You may feel that you need help in transitioning your diet to ensure that you are doing the best for your body and lifestyle. For support with detoxing and dieting,

It's your body! The *best* food gives best results and a healthier, energised body.

The Recipe for Energy

Establish a diet of plenty of fresh vegetables and fruit, preferably eaten raw or near to raw. Then add a little cooked fish and meat if you choose. Avoiding all processed and pre-packaged foods, particularly any with additives, is your number one priority. Things like flavour enhancers, preservatives, emulsifiers, thickeners, and all the other chemicals that those three-digit numbers in the contents/additives list of the packaging represent.

KISS, 'Keep it simple, silly,' and you will be amazed at how well you feel and how you can keep the cost of food down too. Be sure all the fruit and vegetables you consume are as close to ripe as possible when harvested. There's a simple check you can do. Fruits and vegetables have a distinct aroma when properly ripe. When you are doing your pre- purchase inspection, check for this. The produce should have at least some of the aroma of its variety!

When it does, buy it! When it does not, leave it in the store!

Tests have proved that many types of fruit and vegetables develop more than half of their full nutritional benefits during the last four days of their ripening process. The closer to properly ripe the fruit and vegetables are before harvest, the better it is for you. That's what nature intended, and that's how you can be sure you are getting the best nutrients for your well-being. Todays factory farming world does not help.

The important thing to understand is that we really are what we eat. Looking after your body, eating live, fresh, ripe, raw fruit and vegetables enhances that life vitality in you and helps your stomach and bowels to work better for your increased well-being.

Raw Foods versus Cooked Foods

The fact that for perhaps the last five to ten generations, the majority of our food has been cooked, and for many, now all their food is cooked, it does not prove that this is how we should live. We have become addicted to the taste factor in our diets with man-made added *sugar* being a big part of this confusion. Being lazy and not wanting to chew our food as much as we should for the benefit of helping our digestive system work properly is also a concern. Cooking has provided an opportunity to build tastes into our diet that appeal to our senses but are not always beneficial for our bodies. This does not prove that we are alive and healthier as a benefit of all this cooked food but, rather, the opposite; it reinforces the strength and determination of our body's life force to sustain us, regardless of how we mistreat ourselves. Plus this is the major contributing factor to why millions of us are existing in bodies which are carrying around massive toxic loads. Why else do we have societies and medical systems supporting a huge number of people with all sorts of serious health issues and overweight which are getting progressively worse, with no likely improvement in sight?

The aim for each of us should be to live in a healthy, energised, and balanced body, well into old age, after which we simply expire in our sleep to the next world. There are several small communities around the world who are achieving this goal. Make it your aim to follow that precedent. But the important ingredient in achieving this goal is looking after your body in a holistic way as you go through life!

The Importance of Enzymes

Part of our life-force process is enzymes, which are catalysts to all our body's operating systems. They are needed for every chemical reaction that occurs in our body. Without them, no activity would take place. Vitamins, minerals, and hormones are useless without enzymes. Enzymes work in temperatures from freezing up to 118°F. Above that, they quickly become sluggish and over 130°F (47.8°C to 54.5°C) are dead.

Therefore, *any* food you eat that has been heated to above 130°F at any time during its journey from plant to you, has a limited amount of live enzymes. At boiling point, 212 degrees, there will only be *dead* enzymes. As a direct consequence of this fact, you should put all these foods in your 'eat less' category. Now this revelation does challenge lots of long-held social beliefs, all of which are based purely on established habits and without any scientific backing! For you to have the proper balance for your health and vitality, it is essential to eat food that contains live, vital organic elements and nutritional enzymes. All fresh, raw fruits, vegetables, seeds, and nuts provide these essential ingredients, which all work to enhance your well-being.

We are all born with a certain amount of enzymes. That's why it is important to supplement your diet with enzyme-rich raw food. Once you run out of enzymes, your life ends. The lack of enzymes is a primary cause of premature ageing and an underlying cause of degenerative disease and death.

Another important point to be made here is that cooking of most foods increases their acidity and simply adds another factor to this whole pH balance/imbalance story.

Foods You Must Avoid

For your best health, avoid all foods that have added chemicals for flavouring, preserving, thickening, and other ingredients you do not recognise! Especially avoid foods that have ingredients with numbers. Avoid foods which have been tampered with or processed. There is one food I would like to draw your attention to in particular. Although it might be perceived as a natural product with no added chemicals, at the top of the list should be man-made sugar.

Man-Made Sugar—the Sweet Poison!

In his book *Sweet Poison: Why Sugar Makes Us Fat*, David Gillespie provides all the evidence through his inspiring collection of research and statistical facts as to why this is so! It is only during the last 150 years that humanity has had access to sugar in overdose proportions. The world of business has acted on our overwhelming craving to put more sugar into our diet and body. Man-made sugar is in *all* soft drinks; most beers; all pastries, cakes, biscuits, and jams; most breakfast cereals and dessert dishes, and it gets hidden in all sorts of fast foods to keep you coming back for more! It is used extensively in low-fat foods. Plus you will find it in a whole host of other pre-packed foods that would cover the next three pages if listed. You need to check everything for yourself. Our body's natural instinct and response to this dramatic change in sugar supply is to save it as *fat* just in case you might need it tomorrow or next week when you cannot find food. That is the body's instinctive response every time it gets an extra supply of sugar.

That was fine a few centuries back and thousands of years ago, when there was no shop selling food on every corner. Now we can easily find food everywhere in our modern society, thus the epidemic health crisis we are seeing across all our new world societies today. This crisis can, and mostly does, then develop into all sorts of health issues, many for which the medical establishment can then prescribe warfarin and other drugs that all mask the real issue.

If you are one of those overweight people, you must read the above book and *stop* consuming man-made sugar and its substitutes. It will give you all the evidence you need to change your life! Gillespie makes a very real connection between your desire not to exercise when overweight and the real reason why you do not want to exercise. The simple answer is that your body is out of balance with nature's way! Get yourself back in tune with nature's way, and then your body will return to 'normal'. To do this, you simply proceed and apply all the principles of this book for your health and vitality.

Do not, under any circumstances, consider using artificial (man- made) sweeteners as a way of reducing your sugar intake. There is a mass of evidence and results out there that show the effects on you and your body are even worse than genuine man-made sugar.

An Easy Transition to a Healthier Diet

I recommend that you try juices and smoothies to ease your transition into a healthier lifestyle.

Start with changing and experimenting with just one meal a day, preferably breakfast. Get yourself a juicer. Make a fresh vegetable soup, smoothie, or juice from a mixture of vegetables and fruit. Mix a little fruit with it to lighten the taste till you get accustomed. Aim to use 60–70 per cent of vegetables!

For warfarin users, be careful to mix only small amounts of the vegetables high in vitamin K as per the list under the heading 'Foods That Affect Warfarin's Efficacy' in chapter 7.

Use a proper juicing machine that squeezes the liquid from the original fruit and vegetables! You then consume the juice and discard the fibre. This provides a fully fluid and healthy, quickly digested snack or meal. You can try all sorts of food combinations till you arrive at the best combinations to suit your personal preference. Discarding the fibre enables quick digestion. Use a good quality juicer to achieve the best percentage of juice separation from the solids. The Green Power juicer is one that you can rely on as a premium work assistant.

There are several other benefits! If you are having chewing problems, then the juicer has effectively done all the chewing for you. You just need to take your time while consuming the smoothie to allow your saliva sufficient time to mix with the food as you consume it. Also there is a saying, 'Chew your juice and drink your food.' This basically is saying that you need to start the digestion process by making some chewing actions while drinking and that you should chew your food until it is almost liquid to aid digestion! Take your time, sip and savour your meal; it all helps to enable your digestive system to work at its optimum and adds to your nutritional satisfaction. The result is better health and vitality for *you*.

Warfarin users should go cautiously when starting the transition to juice diets. Introduce changes in the types of foods you use gradually over a period of several INR tests. This will ensure that the change in diet is not having too dramatic a change to your INR readings and will allow your warfarin dose to be adjusted if needed.

The main criteria to keep in mind when juicing are:

1. Use only three to five ingredients in each mix you make.
2. Use high–vitamin K vegetables sparingly.
3. Vary the mix often to add variety.
4. Make only sufficient for your immediate use whenever possible.
5. Be sure to have sufficient sweet fruit in each mix to suit your taste preference.

Over time, you will find you can reduce the sweet ingredients as you become accustomed to this new way of treating yourself.

Work your way gradually into this change.

You may feel some resistance to this plan in the first few weeks. This will soon pass, and you will feel real benefits soon after continuing with this new way of living

CHAPTER 7

VITAMINS, MINERALS, AND SUPER FOODS THE VITAMIN K FACTOR & WARFARIN

R eaders are advised that the next 4 pages down to the sub heading **"Herbs and Spices"** is information specific to warfarin users and is of little relevance to other readers so for you other readers feel free to skip these next 6 pages.

Vitamin K and the level or proportion of it circulating in our bodies is a key issue in what this whole warfarin treatment regimen is about. Here are some more insights on the subject for your further understanding and preparedness.

Research into vitamin K over the past twenty years, revealed in the document 'Living with Warfarin', shows and reinforces the benefit of consuming your ideal daily intake of vitamin K. It shows that by consuming the recommended 50 to 150 mcg a day, vitamin K will provide you with increased long-term resistance to a variety of issues that can be caused by lack of this essential vitamin. You may need a little extra warfarin to balance this, but it's a desirable side effect for your overall health. Here's the full explanation and what you can do to help yourself.

There are two types of vitamin K available to us from nature, plus supplements from this New Age world of pharmaceutical development.

K1—principally from green, leafy vegetables as per the list below. K1 breaks down quickly in the body, usually within twelve hours, and does have a substantial effect on INR levels as your daily intake changes, hence the need to be cautious of intake amounts and changes. K2—menaquinone is synthesised by animal tissues and in our body and is found in meat, eggs, and dairy products. Bacteria produce it during digestion and fermentation of foods. K2 lasts up to seventy-two hours in our body and has significantly less effect on INR levels when taken in low-to-moderate doses as a supplement. (It appears difficult to find supply sources of K2.)

Vitamin K is essential in the synthesis of osteocalcin, the hormone that promotes bone formation. Several epidemiological studies have concluded that a vitamin K deficiency (such as that induced by warfarin therapy) and the recommended avoidance of foods with moderate to high vitamin K, causes reduction in bone mineral density and increases the risk of fractures as a direct result. Other studies have shown that the concurrent use of menaquinone (vitamin K2) and vitamin D3 substantially reduce this bone loss and, in some cases, reverse the process to some degree.

There is evidence that the average dietary intake of vitamin K for warfarin users is insufficient to ensure optimum osteocalcin production (for bone strength) and, hence, your recommended daily intake should be increased. Supplementation with vitamin K2. Moderate exercise helps and, combined with an appropriate intake of vitamin D, calcium, magnesium, boron, zinc, and vitamin K (preferably K2), can substantially reduce the risk of bone loss and fractures.

A recent check of my personal bone status reveals the above issue is very real in me and I need to take substantial action as per above to reduce the risk of a hip fracture for myself. Have you been advised of this risk from any other sources? Perhaps you should take note.

The newer anticoagulants, Dabigatran and Rivaroxaban, have different mechanisms of action that do not interact with vitamin K and may be taken with supplemental vitamin K. You may want to look at that alternative to change from warfarin use if your bone density is an issue and your doctors will permit the change.

Vitamin K—the Importance of Having Some Every Day!

From the previous section, we can see the importance of maintaining some daily intake of vitamin K. It is a key factor that the body uses to maintain bone and cardiovascular health. Recent studies have shown that having this small daily intake of 50 to 150 mcg/day actually helps you maintain a more stable INR level. This small dose also helps the body maintain desirable bone health levels and reduce the risk of osteoporosis and related bone fracture risks. Having a low to no daily intake of vitamin K will increase the risk of bone fracture in older people by up to 65 per cent and also compounds the risks of other health issues. Vitamin K also helps protect against blood vessel calcification and coronary heart disease, more reasons it is important to maintain some degree of balance for your ongoing health. It has also been found that moderate amounts of K2 have little effect on INR levels. Vitamin D also adds to this balance. Be sure you are getting your daily fifteen to thirty minutes of sunshine.

If you use warfarin, then you must balance that vitamin K effect on warfarin's work.

The main foods that can affect warfarin efficacy are listed below. Be aware of those vegetables. Use very small amounts of those at the top of the range. When you change your intake of any of those green vegetables from the mid to upper part of the list below, do so progressively over several INR tests so as to ensure your INR stays within range and you have time to adjust your warfarin intake, should that be needed.

Those high in vitamin K increase your blood's clotting ability and reduce the effect of warfarin, proportionate to their mcg level of vitamin K. The higher the mcg number, the more effect that vegetable has on your INR level.

For your best health, this is my perception and understanding from nature's holistic food's point of view. It is far better for your overall health that you have a daily intake of raw foods, including some or all of those below (spread over a weekly or more cycle) in small portions to achieve a good dietary balance. I have found better health by consuming these foods and taking more warfarin to compensate rather than the recommended option of some medical establishments to avoid them all and, hence, miss the nutritional benefit of the added variety these foods provide for my health.

The vegetables listed below have high vitamin K1 levels listed in order of approximate quantities you should eat assuming a mix of four food types from the entire list on any one day. All figures are for *raw* foods.

The gram-size portions quoted below are serving-size amounts to achieve proportionate restricted intake suited for people using warfarin to prevent excessive intake of vitamin K1 while achieving the ideal 100 mcg daily intake and evening out the amounts of each food type for your total serving list.

The portions quoted below in grams (approximate ounces or part ounces, *US* in brackets) are the ideal serving sizes which will provide you with 25 per cent of the ideal maximum daily intake of vitamin K for that food type. Combine or add any four of these foods using the serving size recommended below to meet your daily recommended maximum intake of 100 per cent vitamin K. The list starts with foods of high vitamin K content, hence the small serving size, and works down towards foods with low vitamin K content. Hence the portion sizes increase as you go down the list. All figures are based on raw food values. After cooking, some values may vary.

Foods That Affect Warfarin's Efficacy

For warfarin users, here is a list of leafy green foods that you should eat in limited amounts as per the quantities shown. Take desired maximum serving size with a combined total of any four of the food types below per day to meet maximum vitamin K1 intake limit.

Food Type

Parsley 1g 1⁄29oz
Amaranth leaves 2g 1⁄15oz
Swiss chard 2.5g 1⁄12oz
Dandelion greens 2.7g 1⁄11oz
Kale 2.8g 1⁄10oz
Garden cress 3.5g ⅛oz
Lamb quarters (USA) 3.5g ⅛oz
Spinach 4g ⅐oz
Collards 4.5g ⅙oz
Basil 4.8g ⅙oz
Chicory 7.0g ¼oz
Watercress 8.0g ¼oz
Mustard greens 8.0g ¼oz
Turnip greens 8.0g ¼oz
Sweet potato leaves 8.0g ¼oz
Radicchio 9.0g ⅓oz
Chives 12g ⅖oz
Brussels sprout 13g ½oz
Lettuce (red leaf) 15g ½oz
Lettuce (green leaf) 17g ⅗oz
Lettuce (butterhead) 20g ¾oz
Lettuce (cos and romaine) 20g ¾oz
Lettuce (iceberg) 70g 2.4oz
Broccoli 20g ¾oz
Cabbage 25g ⅞oz
Endive (raw) 30g 1oz

Leeks 42g 1.4oz
Asparagus 55g 2oz
Kiwi fruit (green) 55g 2oz

Other vegetables between 70 and 115 grams per serve (2.4 to 4 oz):

okra, beans
horseradish
rhubarb
alfa seeds (sprouted)
mung beans (sprouted)
cucumbers
capers.

Foods above 115 grams per serve (4 oz):

celery
soybeans (sprouted)
peas
onions
potatoes, pumpkins, and all those not previously mentioned
fruits with higher vitamin K levels (ie grapes).

After the above, the range starts to spread among all other food types, and the vitamin K levels in those are not likely to have any significant effect on one's INR levels.

*   *   *

The herb, St John's wort (*Hypericum perforatum*), often taken for depression, is one which should be avoided completely for other reasons.

Microwaving your food - DO NOT DO IT

Herbs and Spices

There is a vast array of herbs available; almost all of them provide some particular health benefit to aid our coping with and better resistance to a wide array of health issues. Some particular herbs provide real results without the man-made chemical side effects. Because there is no patentable benefit to the financial system, you have to do your own research as to what can work best for you. Make a point to find those particular ones best suited to you and get into the habit of adding a little each day to your diet. Spices add vitality and interest to the whole mix. Enjoy them as part of the experience!

Foods that encourage blood thinning include those known as salicylates. If you are one who is known to be salicylate sensitive, you need to establish your own degree of restriction to these foods. Foods high in salicylates include many spices, most fruits and nuts, plus the following list, which is not in order of high or low content and is, by no means, totally inclusive.

ginger avocado cinnamon
paprika thyme dill
oregano turmeric liquorice peppermint raisins grapes
prunes mango cherries
cranberries blueberries strawberries oranges tangerines

There could be others that could be added to this list. Aspirin is also a salicylate. I personally have had no problem with any of them and have not been able to make any connection to symptoms. (I do not use aspirin and avoid all pain killing drugs as much as possible.) The low pH issue, out of balance small intestine bacteria combined can cause leaky gut syndrome which then spreads to aches in your joints and other issues like ongoing diarrhoea!

Other Vitamins

Sometimes our body needs additional help to allow it to reach optimum health, especially if we have been operating at a low level of health for some time. Also if you tend to be a light eater, foods with a higher level of nutrients can be helpful. Many of us, due to ill health, poor diet, or ageing bodies often benefit from additional support. I am not a nutritionist, but I wanted to provide you with an introduction to the subject of supplementing your diet.

Given our less-than-perfect diets, the mineral-deficient soil in which much of our foods are now grown, monolithic cropping practices used by a large portion of broad-acre agriculture, and the generally less-than-healthy lifestyles many of us live by, it can enhance your well-being to supplement with premium vitamins and minerals and super foods. So read on!

In this age of monoculture farming and mass-produced food, being sure you are getting the full range of all essential vitamins and minerals is almost impossible. Taking a daily allowance of premium-grade nutritional supplements will eliminate this risk for you and ensure you are consuming the full recommended daily requirements by providing those few essential vitamins that may be missing from our mass-produced food supply.

Patients on long-term warfarin therapy are recommended to ensure they get desired daily supplements for the following: vitamins C, D3, and K; magnesium; calcium; potassium; boron; zinc; proline; lysine; and perhaps green tea. These amounts can be achieved from six to seven servings of fresh fruits and vegetables per day. (Patients with kidney issues should seek medical advice first.) If you cannot achieve this daily intake of fresh fruits and vegetables, then you should seriously consider a daily supplement of premium vitamins.

Vitamin B12—A Common Vitamin Deficiency

This is one that often shows when your pH level is out of balance (which for me took several years to figure out, and you may well be having the same confusing learning experience).

It has also been my observation over time that as your body pH level gets out of balance to the acid side, your natural ability to produce your own B12 is substantially diminished, causing all sorts of side effects, to which most mainstream medicos prescribe solutions that only patch or mask the problem. That has been my personal experience and, hence, one of the reasons for writing this book. As you get your pH levels back to a more balanced position, you will find your need for B12 supplements diminishes and, after a time, you become self-sufficient again.

Here's one shortcut to help you restore your B12 to ideal levels.

One of the many symptoms of low B12 levels is acid reflux. B12 is essential for a whole range of functions, and many of the B12 deficiency symptoms are identical to symptoms of other issues, all of which tend to confuse effective diagnosis! Low B12 contributes to the following symptoms: low iron, stomach acid, bloating, thyroid issues, and many more. The most effective forms of B12 supplementation are only available through either stick on patches that you use, every few days, as a spray you use under your tongue or as a monthly direct injection. Perhaps if I had read this book again in 2020 I could have avoided my acid reflux journey' The getting older causes one to forget these tips.

Other symptoms include lethargy, weight loss, anxiety, and depression.

You will be amazed at how many of your health issues may be very directly related to a lack of the very essential vitamin B12 and equally amazed at the lift in your vitality when you begin supplementing your diet. As you age you lose the ability to secrete hydrochloric acid that helps to release vitamin B12 from your food. To further exacerbate the problem it is hard to absorb through the stomach so even if you are eating foods or taking supplements that are rich in vitamin B12 it is unlikely that you are getting enough. You would only absorb around 1 per cent at best from a capsule supplement dose. Studies show that about 80 per cent of vegans or live/raw foodies become B12 deficient and 39 per cent of meat eaters are B12 deficient. Also the type of B12 provided in the capsule form is not the ideal one for us anyway. If you suspect you are deficient, then get tested. The gold standard test is a methylmalonic acid test. Other standard tests may show false results!

Here are some other ways you can treat acid reflux. In most cases, acid reflux is actually caused by your pH level being out of balance. The shortcut cure is a pill that masks the problem but does not help resolve the issue in the long term. A more effective long-term solution is the consumption of a small amount of apple cider vinegar, about 10 to 15 ml mixed with equal to double the volume of water. Drink this once daily before you have your main meal. This gives a boost to acid levels in the stomach and dramatically helps get your stomach rebalanced. You may need to do this for three months or longer until things get back to normal. The B12 solution gives the same result but quicker. Once you get your body fully in tune with the pH-recommended diet and all is going along comfortably, your stomach and small intestine produce your own supply of vitamin B12, thus eliminating the need for further outside supplements of B12! (You may still need to consider your age factor in this and use the spray or patches if you need to.)

Minerals

Many of us are deficient in minerals due to the poor quality of the food we eat and deficient levels in the soil in which our food is grown. The most common are:

1. **Iodine**. This trace mineral is very important to our health, especially our thyroid. It is a crucial ingredient in thyroid health, and the lack of it will lead to hypothyroidism, which

will manifest symptoms such as weight gain, an inability to lose weight, fatigue, elevated blood lipids, hair loss, dry skin, loss of libido, or infertility, to name a few. You can find this mineral in seaweed, seafood, and egg yolks. Older readers in Australia should consider a small supplement of this to your diet as it is deficient in old soils & hence our food supply.

2. **Selenium.** A minor deficiency is common, and the best foods you can eat to counter this are Brazil nuts, wild salmon, lamb, cremini and shiitake mushrooms, turkey, cod, and egg yolks.

3. **Magnesium.** Probably 50 per cent of the population are deficient in this mineral. This is linked to heart disease, asthma, colon cancer, and type 2 diabetes, to name a few. Symptoms include migraines, constipation, restless leg syndrome, and cramping. The best way of getting more magnesium into your body is to eat lots of leafy greens. It is also found in dark chocolate, nuts, and seeds.

Superfoods

There are a few superfoods that supply extraordinary levels of nutrients to our bodies, giving anti-ageing, longevity, and health benefits. A great book to read on the subject is David Wolfe's *Superfoods*. In the meantime, here are a few of my favourite superfoods.

Honey, the Nectar of the Gods!

Honey is the food gathered and made by the world's bee population as part of their work to pollinate flowers for the vast variety of plants around the planet.

Over one third of our modern world food sources rely on the very important work of the honeybee to complete pollination of their flowers and, hence, see the fertilisation process in each and every individual flower triggering the development of that particular plant's fruit, vegetable, or seed.

This interdependence between plants, bees, and us is recognised in the scientific world as vital to both the plants and us, the human race. The work of bees needs all the encouragement and protection we can give them, through all sectors of our scientific, government, farming, and personal worlds! Mankind's interfering and tampering with nature, through the use of pesticides and other chemicals and via genetic engineering, in some instances, is having dramatic and negative effects on the world's bee population. That, in turn, will have negative effects on the amount of food available to us from those plants, which rely on bees for pollination of their flowers to make their life cycle work and produce their seeds, fruits, and vegetables.

Honey is chemically complex, with more than 180 components. Honey provides essential antioxidants, minerals, vitamins, amino acids, enzymes, carbohydrates, and phytonutrients to the body. Honey is totally natural and a highly versatile sweetener, and if still raw, honey will have a whole range of nature's special enzymes that add to your health and well-being. It is the only food source of bees.

There is a whole host of built-in micro supplements that enable bees to live on it without any other food source. The same cannot be said for man-made sugar, as I have already talked about. Studies have shown that natural raw honey may be able to inhibit the effects of toxic substances present in our body. Some especially collected Manuka honey types from Australia and New Zealand have healing properties. A number of food engineers claim that honey is simply the same as sugar, but the reality is much different. It may be high on the fructose scale at around 40 per cent, but nature has built amazing complexity into honey. Honey was the only food found inside the Egyptian pyramids that was still recognisable. What a feat after four thousand years! Also, honey is a fructose-type sugar, which puts it in the 'good' sugar category, and has a low glycemic index value.

Do this simple comparison test for yourself.

Taste and eat a teaspoon of raw honey, preferably direct from a beehive comb. Then taste and eat a teaspoon of sugar. Your taste buds will tell you without doubt which has all the inbuilt energy and positive vibrations from nature. Because honey is a complete food, in its natural state with nothing taken away, your body is satiated. When you have incomplete foods such as man-made sugar, your body recognises that something is missing and seeks the missing parts; hence, you feel the need to eat more. This is one of those important indicators built into your digestive system; it only works with natural whole foods. Try a few different honey flavours and find one you prefer. My favourite is Australian yellow box honey, the product of our native bush gum trees!

Honey! Truly, the nectar of the gods! Do your little bit to support this vital work of our bees and help our food production system in the process! If you use sugar, change to honey where appropriate. Your support for their work will be appreciated. Plus your body will feel and know the difference with all those subtle tastes from nature's garden. Every time you have a teaspoon of honey, think of the thousands of flowers from which the bees collected its components. Then build on that thought in your mind of all those flowers providing this gift from nature's garden to you, which you get to enjoy at that moment! This is my life experience with honey. Honey should only be classed as one of nature's special super foods.

Be aware when you buy your honey that it comes from a respectable reliable honest supplier so you can be sure you are getting the real premium product. In Australia we have a major retail supplier that mostly sell 3rd grade mixed product so check out your supplier's source. The price may give you some guide!

Walnuts!

Walnuts are another of nature's special foods and a specific brain food that benefit your whole body. Science has identified some thirty-five-plus different compounds in walnuts that are all good for the workings of our brain. As we go past middle age and on, it is important to help maintain optimum brain function. Have just one or two kernels a day, and you will feel and know the difference over time. Nuts, in general, are pure, raw, healthy foods straight from nature, with high-protein content as a bonus! If you find the chewing an issue, soak them, break them up, grind them, or mix with other foods in your blender when making drinks.

In fact, soaking nuts is a great idea, as it removes the enzyme inhibitors and allows the nut to begin the sprouting process. This releases more nutrients for your body to absorb. Also, do not assume that the nuts you buy are raw. Many have been subject to an assortment of processes to satisfy 'regulations'. If the nuts cannot be germinated, that is your answer.

Other Tree Nuts

Macadamia, pecan, almond, and some others all have special high-nutritional value, plus the benefits of being highly transportable and storable at room temperature for months without degrading. They are great snack foods with good protein content. Ideal to add to your school or work lunch!

Brazil nuts deserve special mention because of their high concentration of selenium, which is commonly deficient in some parts of the world food supplies. Also, this helps boost our natural in-body ability to produce our own supply of co-enzyme Q10, important for our heart's health.

Coconut—That 'Different' Big Nut

Classified as a functional food because of its range of contents, including meat, juice, milk, fibre, and oil with healing properties! The coconut has fed and nourished populations around the world for thousands of years. Have a tablespoon of pure coconut oil with your meals to give a major energy boost and reduce fat accumulation. Use it on your toast or bread instead of butter and/or margarine. Use it as your cooking oil instead of the other recommended options!

Real-life experience doing this has proved for many people you can be more energised and loose a little weight as you go because of the energising and metabolising properties of coconut oil, plus have the added benefit of being in tune with nature's way by using this proven staple food for your well-being and benefit.

Other Nuts

Note the root vegetable type, such as peanuts, fit into a totally different category with not all the benefits of the nuts described above.

Sprouted Grains!

After a seed has started its growing cycle, the evidence shows the nutritional benefit increases five- to tenfold. You can buy grains and seeds ready sprouted in small quantities, for which you pay a substantial premium, or you can get your own seeds/grains and sprout them at home. Grains generally have a low pH factor, but after the sprouting process begins, the pH changes to positive! Sprouting provides a massive boost to the nutritional value of nuts and seeds and all the natural energy that comes forth as part of nature's new life process. You get this *ten* times the nutritional and energy benefit from consuming sprouted grains in all forms when compared to raw, dry grain as used in flour, etc. Eat them raw, juice them, or mix them with other foods in your blender. The lift in your well-being will amaze you, plus you get the full benefit of the grain as a whole food with all its components included, as distinct from the partial food you get in flour and bread, biscuits, cereals etc. Some medium and larger seed varieties tend to have a small percentage of seeds that do not absorb water and sprout. These seeds can remain quite hard on your teeth, so you may find it desirable to sieve these out after your batch has sprouted before consuming your newly sprouted and growing food.

Other Special Foods

Chia seeds. This is the superfood of the Aztec culture and available from most health food stores. Chia has the highest plant-based source of omega-3 and fibre, plus protein and that elusive vitamin B12. All eight essential and nine non-essential amino acids are included for good measure. Because of the really small seed size, chia is best added as a sprinkle over your salads and other prepared foods or tossed into your mixed-vegetable dish and eat fresh. Add a level dessert spoon of seeds to a glass of water, stir for a minute or two, and drink before it starts to gel. This will provide extended energy to your meals and the feeling of being full, thus reducing your desire to snack and helping to lose weight if needed.

To make a chia seed pudding, blend cashews, honey, water and a few drops of vanilla essence. Stir in some chia seeds. Pour into a glass dish and leave to set. Chia oil extract is also available with its high concentration of omega-3 ALA. Be sure to use only 100 per cent certified pure chia from sources that produce premium-grade product. Avoid seeds grown in China.

Açai berry. A fruit from the Amazon basin available from a variety of producers in a wide range of forms from partly dried to fully processed and powdered. Take a look and make your personal choice. Google *açai berry* and see for yourself. **Cacao.** This is one of the raw materials from which chocolate is made. It can be purchased as a powder, a solid nib, or in butter form from health food stores and online. Use it to make your own healthy chocolates, puddings, cakes, and drinks. **Aloe Vera.** From the aloe vera plant we get a whole range of products from juice to drink to creams, powders, and more. All bring well-proven health and other benefits to us! There is a wide variety of producers and specialist suppliers to choose from. Check it out at your local health food store or google *aloe vera* and see for yourself.

CHAPTER 8

EXERCISE AND MOVE YOUR BODY

Breathe

Get into the habit of spending five minutes when you wake up and again in the evening breathing in deeply through your nose, holding for five seconds, then breathing out through your mouth. Oxygen is our most vital and most instantly demanded nutrient for the body. We can only survive for five minutes without it. By spending this time fully oxygenating your body, you will find that within ten to fifteen minutes, you will feel better. Any pain issues tend to be reduced, and all your body's functions are improved because of the increased oxygen. People doing passive occupations should make a particular point to focus on this. It is so easy and simple, plus the benefits come quickly!

Move More The Basis for Your Whole Body to Work Properly

Every time we move, we use up some of the kilojoules (or calories) that are in the food that we eat. The kilojoules that we do not use up will be stored as fat. 'Move more' reminds us that we need to balance the energy (kilojoules) that we take in with the energy we use. We eat daily, so we need to be active daily. Action was always part of our daily routine until the machine and computer age changed all that. Be proactive and ensure you get your daily exercise for your body and mind's benefit.

Add plenty of what are classed as non-active exercise habits to your daily pattern or ritual. These simple activities have a dramatic effect on your well-being if you have been in the habit of remaining motionless for long periods of sitting. Make this change your norm from now on. Do any one of these simple ten- to thirty-second activities several times in every hour of your previously motionless time:

- Stand up, take a few steps, perhaps have a drink of water.
- Go to your window and look at the view for ten seconds.
- Get up and say hello to someone around the corner.
- Take a comfort stop and stretch on the way.
- Stand and touch your toes.
- Walk clockwise around the room.
- Walk the opposite way around the room.

The point here is to get in the habit of moving your body several times in every hour!

Add these actions to your day; make it part of the norm in addition to your real exercise routine. NASA has done research on this and found real benefits in these simple short breaks. Take your routine back a few generations when movement was an integral part of every hour in your waking day! We do have all the benefits of our new technology age, but to be sure of enjoying it in your healthy body, you must make this conscious decision to live deliberately and work at the things your body needs for optimum health! The older we get, the more important these simple movement habits are!

Also, our body's lymph duct and gland system, having no pump of its own, depends totally on the pumping action of our muscles to circulate our body waste fluids through this network. By expanding and contracting one's muscles, this action contributes to the effective flow of body wastes through our lymph duct network. This workout enables our body to clear toxins away from our cells and enhance our general health. This is important when you think that much of today's diseases are exacerbated by a build-up of toxins and wastes in our system.

You will observe some pain throughout your body as you start to exercise after a period of no activity. This is your body telling you that all this crap and waste build-up is on the move through your lymph network. After you have spent time exercising, you will feel better.

Buy yourself an exercise machine, or move the one you have and put it in the lounge room in front of the TV. Get on it and get exercising as you watch your favourite show. Your visitors may think having this machine in your living room a bit odd, but seeing you achieve better health will inspire them! You will be more inclined to do your exercise while you are being entertained and distracted from thinking about how your body is feeling. Or better still, listen to your favourite music or DVD from the positive people listed in chapter 11. Try it—you will be inspired by the combination. Drink plenty of water as you exercise!

Remember, it's your body, and you must use all the ways you can to keep in tune.

CHAPTER 9

LIVING DELIBERATELY

Make it your focus to think through your lifestyle and develop and act on a positive plan. If you just go with the flow, you often end up being a victim of your own subconscious negative paradigms and inbuilt animal-like instinctive reactions to events. Ways of thinking and reacting that were learned as a child often do not serve us in a positive way. It's your choice. Make your own decisions as to what is best for you and your body instead of going with the flow of general consensus on food and lifestyle.

Your Mind You Have the Ability to Control Your Thoughts

We become what we think about most of the time. Here are a variety of insights and connections, which show and reinforce this most profound and basic point of where we can *choose* to operate from. We live in a world where we can, and mostly are, being constantly bombarded with masses of information . . . most of it negative!

It is up to you to choose what's important and beneficial for your health and well-being then focus and act on that information to the exclusion of the negative stuff. When you do that, you will find a whole host of improvements and changes just seem to happen in your life.

Thomas Troward, in his book *The Hidden Power*, said, 'If thought power is good for anything, it is good for everything. We must see and use thought as the preamble to everything.'

With the same idea, U. S. Anderson said, 'If we fully realise that thought causes all, we will know there's never any limits that we ourselves do not impose. Thought is the preamble to everything. If it can produce one thing, it can produce anything. For what's to hinder it? Nothing can stop us from thinking . . . nothing.'

Nelson Mandela proved after twenty-five years of internment that no one could cause him to think something he did not want to think. Now play with this for a moment. We think into form. We create pictures in our minds. Listen to what he says here: 'It is true that to think is to form. If so, do we not see that our limitations are formed in precisely the same manner and same way as our expansions or our wins? Many of us think that conditions outside our thoughts have power over us and we think power into them!' Equally, you can choose to do the opposite and get control of—and for—yourself.

Now I know when you're working on some kind of a project, maybe you're looking at some condition or circumstance and thinking you can't do it because of that. You're thinking power into that condition or circumstance. Kick it out of the way. Understand thought creates all. You are a created being; you can think.

Spend four or five minutes and play with that idea.
Thought creates limitations.
Thought creates wins.
Make up your mind you're going to think wins all day long.

You're not going to put any thought power into conditions or circumstances around you that restrict you.

To give you a simple view of what benefits you and what does not, divide your daily activities into two categories:

1. the thoughts and actions which benefit and work for you
2. the thoughts and actions which tend to produce negative or no results for you.

Get into the habit of applying more energy, and focus towards the thoughts and actions that work for you and show positive results. It is important to fully come to understand the importance of this and how one must apply it in life for the best outcome. We have three levels of being on the thought level, namely emotional, mental, and spiritual, with only one level in the physical!

All of the first three are interconnected to your physical. There is this constant interaction between the mind and body. 'Do not allow your emotional self to sweat the small stuff, be aware that in the bigger picture EVERYTHING is small stuff' Nelson Mandela.

How you react to the small stuff mostly sets the limit as to where you settle on your achievement levels in life. The choice is yours every time. Is the issue that is currently on your mind worth getting excited or frustrated about? Excitement tends to build positive results. Frustration and anger build negative results. Think through this every time you have the choice and apply the action/reaction that will give you the benefits!

The physical universe, as perceived by the body, sends messages to the mind. The mind interprets these perceptions according to past experiences and beliefs, channelling signals for the body to react in ways that seem appropriate based on subconscious beliefs and paradigms. For example, if your mind believes that it is inevitable to fall sick, it will channel a signal to the body, and the body will display symptoms of the illness, eventually leading to you becoming ill. This whole concept and reality is closely bound with our deepest ideas and subconscious paradigms about ourselves, life, and the nature of disease and health. You can just as easily be sending conscious signals to yourself of being healthy and happy and achieve that result. It is your conscious choice of which thought path you follow! Be aware that often, many beliefs have been passed to us by parents and peers. Take a serious look at your beliefs and ask if they serve you in a beneficial way, or if they are really just subconscious paradigms that you let control your life often with negative 'comfort zone' results.

Wow. Spend some time getting your head around all that, and get control of your life! To help us fully develop with this preferred way of thinking and living, we all need a mentor and coach. Does the above idea of getting control of your life appeal to you? Then you should connect with a group or program where you learn how to apply *results that stick* in your life. It's in your best interest to connect with your own personal coach and mentor or group of like-minded people where you can learn, encourage, and support each other. We have the ability, through focused and directed conscious thought, to overcome those subconscious paradigms and take real control of our physical well-being. There are countless examples of people who have achieved this control.

You can be one of them!

Your Psychology!

I quote you, Bob Proctors, your insight on the subject: 'Authors that really changed my life were Napoleon Hill and then Earl Nightingale.' Now *This is Earl Nightingale* is a phenomenal book. Let me share something with you that Earl wrote. He said, 'We live in a world of words. We have a word for everything, and some of these names and labels mean a great deal to us. Words such as love, happiness, success, achievement, joy. All describe conditions which all of us want. But there is one word which controls all of them and which will bring us all of these things, or keep us from getting any of them.'

Ask yourself if you know what that word is. Earl Nightingale referred to it as a magic word.

It's *attitude.*

Do you see? If we have the wrong attitude, we distort everything we see! Everything that comes into our life is distorted! When we have the right attitude, we see clearly. We improve everything. We build rapport with people. Attitude, as Earl Nightingale described it, is a condition of bearing as indicated via our thoughts, our feelings, and our actions. It's everything about us. This power flows into our consciousness, and we choose our mind's pictures. We get emotionally involved with those pictures, and that's what causes us to act. And that's what attitude is. It's the energy that's leaving us that's going out into the universe. And the universe, operating by law, sends it back. We send good energy out and good will come back; bad energy will attract bad energy. Your attitude makes the difference. You can have all those beautiful things—love, happiness, achievement—when you have, and apply, the right attitude.

I'm going to ask you to sit and think for four or five minutes and then make up your mind that you're going to have the best attitude you can possibly have all day long. You'll be glad you did.

Almost all successful people work with mentors to help them, develop, learn, and stay focused. Then direct their energy into successful results. Here's your opportunity to connect with people who have a proven track record of success.

Here's your chance to break out from your existing mediocre life results pattern!

When you choose to apply the above insights, you must use total here & now focus on what you are doing so that you can get the best outcome that will work for you.

Our bodies are absolutely amazing. Our dominant mind vibrations are expressed, by law, as emotions which subsequently lead us to into actions that take us towards our current results. We decide the nature of these vibrations, whether they are of a poverty or prosperity frequency. Take a holistic approach to developing and caring for your mind and body. Treat both of them with particular attention. We are essentially formed of pure energy which needs to circulate, just like blood, oxygen, and money. Being mindful that we only have one body, take excellent care of it. Don't let your body become blocked with stale, negative energy. Shake it up, and let the good stuff flow through you. Do yourself a favour and release the stuff that no longer serves you. You know what it is. This will create great harmony, which when done consistently can only grow, and you will become the better person. You and your body will appreciate it.

If the people you mix with are part of the negative problem in your life then either work to help them change or change your social group, change jobs, move to a new city or suburb.

Attitude is everything! Attitude is defined as your thoughts, feelings, and actions. When you visualise yourself via your conscious mind being in control of your subconscious mind and your physical body, this becomes the obvious way to live. The conscious mind expresses itself via the medium of thought. Work on your subconscious through the medium of feelings and emotions, and the body responds through physical action! Aligning these three parts of your personality will see an 'improved' you.

You will no longer be reacting to situations and environments that life puts your way.

You will be responding to them.

No more 'knee-jerk' reactions.

You will go through a thought process.

You will stop and think how to best work through each situation.

You will then find yourself better equipped to make the appropriate action that is required.

Your perception will shift.

You will be able to see things not just from one point of view.

Integration between your belief and your behaviour is known as *praxis*, where you act upon the very same beliefs that you have intellectually!

Many people believe in something but do not act accordingly. Examine your beliefs, and then live them, act them.

Not only set the example, *be* the example!

Attitude is a beautiful thing once all three components are in sync. It's something everyone should be constantly working towards.

In some of us, this attitude thing is being controlled by negative perceptions of events which we experience as children or perhaps some really traumatic event or thing after that.

Think through your responses to events around you and recognise your automatic subconscious reaction for what it is. When you understand that and know how to better respond, you can change your life!

Use the one gift that we are given above all others in nature: the ability to make conscious decisions which override animal instinct. Make it your passion from now on to get as healthy as you can, so life becomes the joyous experience it should be for us all. Move towards being tuned into health and vitality by applying all the knowledge you can from those sources representing health, vitality, and wellness. Then only connect with the sickness industry when you really need to. Your emotional guidance system will give you the feelings and reinforcement for your positive actions. Make connections with people who focus on wellness as their daily routine. Being in a social network you like and enjoy is good for your mind and body.

Your Fears and Facing Them!

A big part of the learning process in helping you understand your fears to learn as much about the things you fear and why. In most instances, you will find that through your learning, you will come to understand that your mixed thought process is blocking you. This can be described as your terror barrier. As you understand this, you come to know you have a choice. Let the fear control you, or learn that the fear can be overcome, and you can choose to override that fear and establish a pattern of behaviour that serves you in a positive way, thus enabling you to get real control of it and in your life.

All our spiritual leaders throughout history have taught these insights. It's up to you to connect and apply the learning. This phrase best sums up your options here: If you think you can, you can. If you think you cannot, you can't.

Henry Ford put the same idea in this context: Whether you think you can or you can't, either way you are right. It's your choice. You choose which path you prefer to follow. It will dictate your results!

1. To live in a world where you are afraid to look over the edge in case you fall off—being afraid to go outside your comfort zone in case you see something that will require you to make a decision! Perhaps even having to consider whether your perception of things is the right one, and if it is serving you in a beneficial way or otherwise! It's your choice to live in your inner version of hell.

2. Or take the positive path and build your own inner heaven—grasp this world of expanded understanding where anything is possible.

   Now take action and get on with your life and enjoy the journey as you go!

Have a serious think about those last few paragraphs and chapters.

Do you have a firm grasp on the whys and wants of your life, or are you being controlled by a bunch of subconscious paradigms? Old beliefs, which developed in your subconscious for reasons that you now do not have any memory of, all of which were developed by negative events in your distant childhood or a time of some major negative life experience. Events and experiences that you could 'reframe' in your mind, allowing you to have a different set of beliefs. With careful attention and understanding of those perceptions, you can change and make life better for yourself!

What you think has a direct effect on your physical body, negatively or positively affecting your acid–alkaline balance. How you communicate with and respond or react to people can also impact on this. The book *Tired of Being Tired* by Jesse Lynn Hanley and Nancy De ville provides a list of acid-forming habits and some other relevant insights

Acid-Making Habits

- anger, rage, complaining, nagging, pessimism
- fear, anxiety, envy, obsessive jealousy, gossip, and backbiting
- harmful emotions and dreams of revenge
- lack of sleep, shallow breathing, and holding your breath
- lack of exercise
- being selfish
- poor communication habits which lead to tensions with other people
- overwork—mostly the mental type
- worry and fretting about all sorts of things, most of which never happen!

Alkaline-Forming Habits

- optimism
- rest—naps, fun, play
- sleep
- fresh air
- laughter
- contentment and happiness
- loving and being loved
- positive communication habits with everyone (which makes us all feel better)
- giving and sharing
- breathing deeply
- exercise.

Somewhere inside each of us is this inbuilt desire to know ourselves. By focusing and building on positive ways of getting on in life, as described here, you too can develop a better connection and insight into that inner smouldering desire, which through life continues to consume the enquiring mind for the answer. Having a positive approach to life allows broader understanding and insight to develop and grow within. This then develops into that real inner strength of getting a better grasp of knowing your inner self, being comfortable and contented within one's self. Take yourself through this journey to see and feel the benefits in your life.

When we change the way we think, we change our lives. What most people do not understand is how powerful our thinking is and how connected it is in our health and well-being.

You can literally think yourself into any situation in life, be it positive, healthy, wealthy, and happy or the opposite. It's your choice!

You control your thoughts! Your thoughts control your actions and results!

CHAPTER 10

THE HEALTH AND WELL-BEING BENEFITS!

What the Application of the Knowledge Learned in This Book Has Done for Me!

By now, you will well and truly have come to know my degree of excitement gained from being able to apply in my life all the ways to enhance my health as discussed throughout this book. Add to that the pleasure gained to be able to share this empowering knowledge with *you*. Here is a collection of the current everyday benefits my seventy five-year-old body enjoys because of this knowledge and my application of it!

More Energy

The first big lift was when I started drinking energised water. Overnight, my sleep pattern went from ten hours and waking up feeling tired to seven hours of sleep and waking up wanting to get out of bed and get into enjoying life and doing things. People have noticed my lift in vitality and energy. The energised and reduced surface tension of this water promotes better circulation and warming/cooling to every extremity of my body. That feeling, hot or cold, is not the issue, it was because of the better circulation around my body. It's as if the energised water cleans the 'porridge' out of one's blood, allowing my whole system to work better!

No Illness

My lifetime of ongoing sinus congestion problems has simply just dried up and gone away almost completely. Being attacked by every cold and flu bug going around is no longer a major concern! Plus, if a sniffle does develop, it clears up within a day or two.

Asthma and Hay Fever Gone

Having ongoing congestion coming up from my lungs and it being treated as asthma without any long-term solution has now stopped happening! Being stricken with hay fever and other allergies to pollens and dust has dramatically diminished. The result? My need to use asthma medication is now down by 50 per cent and more. The chemicals used in these asthma inhalers also add to the acid overload on the body, another reason for you to be working on balancing your overall pH level.

Aching Joints gone

As the combined workings of pH raising and enhanced intestine bacteria levels generally improve my health all the aches & pains from my hips, knees & ankle joints have simply vanished. Saving me lots of money on the health food pills I was buying to fix those aches. Plus walking becomes a joy again!

Gout issues gone

Gout, that other 'acid build-up' issue, has also bugged me from time to time. The acid effect of warfarin on the body helps to increase the build up of Uric acid. Statistics show warfarin users get more gout issues. Taking totally nature based herbal supplements has helped clear uric out of my body. See references at the book last page, for the supplier of herbal products. Another fix that works to help your body expel uric acid is too wear a pure copper finger ring or wrist band. The minute amount of copper adsorbed through your skin helps your body clear the acid build up. It has worked for me!

Consistency of Results from My INR Test

Since becoming comfortable and balanced with the improvements in my health as described through this book, my INR readings at each regular blood test have been much more even and consistent. This means fewer tests at the maximum time between tests of six weeks. This allows one to feel much more comfortable and at ease with the whole regular INR-checking process and with less expense and interruption to one's life. This is backed by research documented by Hans R. Larsen which reinforces the benefit of consuming your ideal daily vitamin K as a support for this action.

Pure Water Builds Better Health

After drinking only quality filtered water for most of the second decade of tis century. With a break for 2-3 years when my water ph changing device died as described earlier and getting a new one a few weeks ago. I found that for the first year plus my desire to drink more water amazed me. Four to five pints a day (two litres and more) was my normal intake. Then after two years of consuming this good, clean water and the cleaning and enhanced health effects it has helped with for my body, I now find my consumption has slowed to two to three pints a day. I feel healthier and better than I have for many years! Again that was 2013, now in 2023 and after being through the traumas of the past 2 -3 years & having my new water ionizer working I'm back to the top again.

All the above health benefits and perhaps a few others have come together for me so that I now feel healthier and *happier* than I have for *decades*. Follow the lead here, and that can be your result too!

Strive to have all your mind and body in optimum health, and then you find that you can expand your focus and your other important goals in life with ease. It lets you put fun and excitement into life.

My Challenge to You!

First you need to buy yourself a personal pH test kit and get accustomed to using it. Second, have your own pH-positive water- filtering system. Now you are ready! The test here is for you to simply carry on your normal life until you next have some form of health issue like a cold or flu or something worse, perhaps even something for which you may feel the desire to get some antibiotics to help overcome this bout of sickness. As this feeling of un-wellness overcomes you, you now place all your focus and attention on breathing, drinking, and eating your pH- positive diet, you will find within a very short time that your body is able to heal itself very effectively. The key point here is that when you live with a higher body pH range in the zone where nature intends your body to work best as your norm, this dramatically enhances your resistance and body's ability to resist all these bugs that attack you from time to time.

Once you have seen and felt this result for yourself, you will have an inner understanding and belief which is stronger than any sales story heard or read from an outside source such as me. The proof for what I have just said comes from my experiences described in this book, plus the testimonials that can be found through all the other books recommended throughout this work and many others.

In the event that your health issue requires major support from the mainstream medical world, then you should use all the help you can get from them. The key point here is that this raised pH factor will speed your healing process regardless of what other aid you use.

To Conclude

Simply live positively, eating and drinking pH-positive food and water, which all combine to build your best possible positive life experience! Have you found some benefit from these pages? Take your time to apply these insights.

Make it a priority to come back and read this whole book in a week and again in a month. Then use the relevant parts as your reference guide until this becomes your normal way of living. Apply what works and what you want to work for you! Keep doing it till the benefits show through in your life.

What can help you achieve your aspirations in life – learn & understand these points

- Why things develop and work the way they do.
- Question and develop better understanding of those workings.
- Apply those insights to make it all work to the best of one's abilities and achieve the best outcome for everyone involved.
- learned that my ability to manage people was best limited to small groups
- Figuring out where you fit on that management scale helps you know where is your spot
- The importance of having and applying a good, efficient, and effective ongoing plan.
- The understanding that when all the rules change because of things outside your control, you need to come to terms with that and then establish a new way to get along in life.

- Know that in life the ultimate rule of natural law applies, which is best described by that old Chinese proverb 'Get yourself in order first and all the other things in life will trend in a better direction from there'.
- Being aware of the fact that people's motivations are often controlled by their learned lifetime subconscious patterns and paradigms (which sometimes make a lot of sense and for others, sometimes, no sense at all even to the individual concerned).
- Having learned on numerous occasions that the perceptions,
- diagnoses, and attitudes of many other 'experts' is not always directed or motivated towards my/your best interests.
- If your skills and knowledge cannot provide the answer, then source someone else who has the required abilities to achieve the desired result. Henry Ford used that extensively!
- A lifetime paradigm developed in my early childhood of always wanting to be helpful, which is a major part of my motivation for writing and publishing this work.
- The ultimate inbuilt desire in all of us to want to feel and live healthy.

Outside-the-Box Health Aides

Premium-grade factory-made colloidal silver is the number-one product that deserves special mention here. It is used extensively throughout the mainstream medical world in bandages to treat burn victims. There is no other substance like it that will kill all 650 of the various bugs, bacteria, viruses, and fungi which are bad for our health. A colloidal silver and water solution of ten to thirty parts per million will kill all of those species within ten minutes when they are immersed in that solution. Yet it has no negative effect on all the 'good bacteria', on which we depend to support and aid our digestive system! So why are we being discouraged from using this product? The hip pocket nerve factor of the medical industry and Big Pharma vested interests is the answer, as discussed in chapter 3.

Mix three parts aloe vera gel with one part colloidal silver solution and you have a premium-grade gel for external use. Google *aloe vera products* for more information.

If you have found benefit from this work, please take the time to help spread the message here. Tell your friends.

I wish you good health, and may life go well for you!

ACKNOWLEDGEMENTS

To these people, who have all helped and inspired me to write this book:

- Tracey Burnett, CHHC, ADDP

- Ann Wood, FSBT, Dip RSA

REFERENCES

- U. S. Anderson. Three magic words

- Bharti Vyas and Suzanne Le Quesne, *The pH Balance Diet*

- www.easyph.com.au

- R. French, 'The Foundation of Balanced Nutrition: Our Acid–Alkaline Status', *Natural Health and Vegetarian Life* (Summer 2006/07)

- David Gillespie, author of *Sweet Poison: Why Sugar Makes us Fat*

- Grander water. Aust, Eng, USA

- Dr Steven Gundry M D the importance correct small intestine bacteria

- Iherb.com suppliers of nature based herbal products & more

- Jesse Lynn Hanley and Nancy De ville. *Tired of Being Tired*

- Napoleon Hill Earl Nightingale Positive thinking & *attitude*

- Gillian McKeith, *You Are What You Eat* (Melbourne: Penguin, 2004)

- Nelson Mandela. Don't sweat the small stuff

- Masaru Emoto, and Wilson Bentley on Water Memory chapter

- 7-16 dow

- Medicaldaily.com microwave concerns Microwaves Are Bad For You

- Harry Palmer, founder and author of *Living Deliberately*

- Bob Proctor. Positive thinking coach

- Steptohealth.com microwave's safety

- Thomas Troward *The Hidden Power*

- Vegsource.com

- Vevor water ionizer. by Vevor .com

- Neale Donald Walsch, *When Everything Changes, Change Everything*

- David Wheeler, DC, and Nora Kosztolanyi, MA, *Water Empowerment for Life.*

- David Wolfe, *Superfoods*

- Dr Robert O. Young, PhD, and Shelley Redford Young, *The pH Miracle*

- youtube.com

The End

Milton Keynes UK
Ingram Content Group UK Ltd.
UKHW012133131223
434271UK00003B/45